PATRICK HOLFORD AND JEROME BURNE

THE

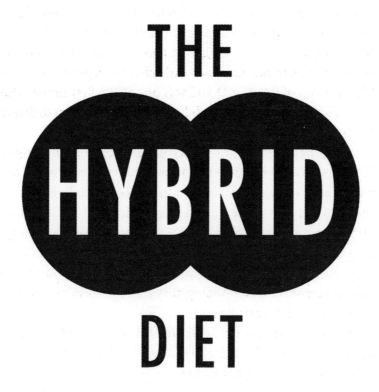

HYBRID

DIET

Your body thrives on two fuels

boost your energy and get leaner and healthier by alternating fats and carbs

piatkus

PIATKUS

First published in Great Britain in 2019 by Piatkus

1 3 5 7 9 10 8 6 4 2

Copyright © Patrick Holford and Jerome Burne 2019

The moral right of the author has been asserted.

With the exception of pages 13, 238 and 262,
internal images © Hollow Earth Ltd 2019

A CIP catalogue record for this book
is available from the British Library.

ISBN 978-0-349-41944-2

Typeset in Minion by M Rules
Printed and bound by CPI Group (UK) Ltd, Croydon, CR0 4YY

Papers used by Piatkus are from well-managed forests
and other responsible sources.

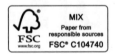

Piatkus
An imprint of
Little, Brown Book Group
Carmelite House
50 Victoria Embankment
London EC4Y 0DZ

An Hachette UK Company
www.hachette.co.uk

www.improvementzone.co.uk

Important Note
This book is not intended as a substitute for medical advice
or treatment. Any person with a condition requiring medical help
should consult a qualified medical practitioner or suitable therapist.

WHAT HYBRID DIETERS SAY

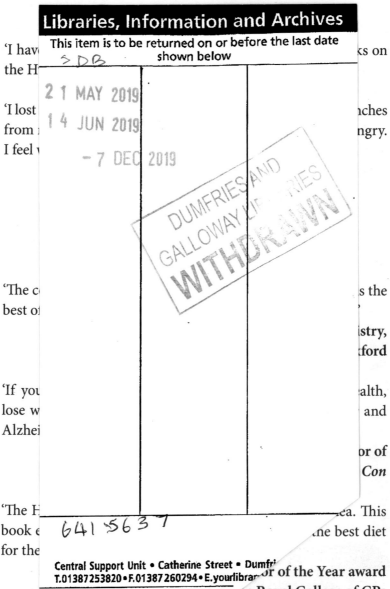

'I hav   ks on
the H

'I lost   iches
from   ngry.
I feel

'The c   s the
best o

                                                          istry,
                                                          tford

'If you   alth,
lose w   and
Alzhei

                                                          or of
                                                          Con

'The H   ea. This
book   ne best diet
for the   or of the Year award
                                        he Royal College of GPs

'Original and provocative. In a world where there seems to be no middle ground, this book dares to suggest that maybe we don't have to choose between fats or carbs but eat real food to accommodate both.'

Dr Zoe Harcombe, nutritionist

'A thoughtful, intelligent, highly informative and practically useful contribution to the seemingly intractable debate on what constitutes a healthy diet.'

Joanna Blythman, award-winning food writer

'This book couldn't be more timely with the obesity and diabetes spiral at an all-time high. A versatile and accessible solution for anyone who's struggled with weight loss or low energy – essential reading.'

Robert Verkerk, founder of Alliance for Natural Health

'Patrick Holford and Jerome Burne are superb communicators and their writings are soundly based on the scientific and medical literature and very much at the forefront of nutritional medicine.'

Emeritus Professor David Smith, University of Oxford

Patrick Holford BSc, DipION, FBANT, NTCRP is a leading spokesman on nutrition in the media, specialising in the field of mental health. He is the author of over 30 books, translated into over 20 languages and selling several million copies worldwide, including *The Optimum Nutrition Bible, The Low GL-Diet Bible, Optimum Nutrition for the Mind* and *Food is Better Medicine than Drugs.*

Patrick started his academic career in the field of psychology. He then became a student of two of the leading pioneers in ortho-molecular medicine and psychiatry – the late Dr Carl Pfeiffer and Dr Abram Hoffer. In 1984 he founded the Institute for Optimum Nutrition (ION), an independent educational charity, with his mentor, twice Nobel prizewinner Dr Linus Pauling, as patron. ION has been researching and helping to define what it means to be optimally nourished for the past 32 years and is one of the most respected educational establishments for training nutri-tional therapists. At ION, Patrick was involved in groundbreaking research showing that multivitamins can increase children's IQ scores – the subject of a *Horizon* documentary in the 1980s. He was one of the first promoters of the importance of zinc, antiox-idants, essential fats, low-GL diets and homocysteine-lowering B vitamins and their importance in mental health and Alzheimer's disease prevention.

Patrick is founder of the Food for the Brain Foundation and director of the Brain Bio Centre, the Foundation's treatment centre that specialises in helping those with mental issues ranging from depression to schizophrenia. He is in the Orthomolecular Medicine Hall of Fame and is an honorary fellow of the British Association of Nutritional Therapy, as well as a member of the Nutrition Therapy Council and the Complementary and Natural Healthcare Council. He is also Patron of the Irish and South African Association of Nutritional Therapy.

Jerome Burne is an award-winning medical and health journalist who, over the last 20 years, has been writing for most of the UK nationals about the latest developments in health and cutting-edge research. He is co-author of *Food is Better Medicine than Drugs*, with Patrick. He was an early champion of probiotics and higher doses of vitamin D and was one of the first in the UK to write about epigenetics – the ability of the environment to directly affect genes.

Jerome has queried the benefits of the widespread prescription of cholesterol-lowering statins to people without heart disease and was one of the first UK journalists to cover the links between the SSRI drugs and suicide in children. He wrote one of the first features investigating the excessive and ineffective prescribing of antipsychotic medication to elderly patients with dementia and was consultant on the 2010 *Panorama* programme on the slow official response to the finding that the diabetes drug Avandia raised the risk of heart disease.

He writes regularly for the *Daily Mail* Good Health pages and edits a blog at HealthInsightUK.org, which promotes a lifestyle approach to health and treatment.

To Gill (Pyrah), my witty and wonderful partner and most incisive critic

Jerome

To Gaby (Holford) for taking care of everything while I vanished down this rabbit hole

Patrick

Contents

Acknowledgements   xi
Guide to Abbreviations and Measures   xiii
Introduction   xv

Part 1

Fat for Fuel   1

1. The High Fat Ketone Revolution   3
2. High Fat, Low Carb Reverses Diabetes   15
3. The High Fat Cancer Hope   23
4. About Turn on High Fat and Heart Disease   34
5. Eat Fat to Lose Weight   42
6. Your Brain Needs Fat   49

Part 2

Slow Carbs Rule   59

7.   Not All Carbs Are Created Equal   61
8.   The Low GL Diet Reverses Diabetes   74
9.   Slow Carbs Win for Weight Loss   84
10. Slow Carbs and Heart Disease   94
11. The High Carbs Cancer Connection   104
12. Slow Carbs Boost Mood and Memory   110

Part 3

Dual Fuel Advantages 117

13. Meet Your Lean, Mean Energy Machine 119
14. Switching on Autophagy: The Cellular Clean-up 132
15. The Value of Intermittent Fasting and Exercise 137
16. Breaking Sugar, Carb and Stimulant Addiction 146
17. Going Hybrid Makes Evolutionary Sense 158
18. Switching: Why, When and How? 173

Part 4

The Hybrid Diet 179

19. Good Fats 181
20. Fruit and Veg: Common Ground 193
21. Don't Exceed Your Protein Needs 204
22. The High Fat Phase 217
23. Slow Carb Phase 235
24. Going Hybrid for Vegetarians, Vegans
    and Pescatarians 260
25. Hybrid Support Micronutrients 270
26. Biohacking Your Ketone/Glucose Balance 284

Part 5

Hybrid Diet Menus and Recipes 301

27. High Fat Phase Breakfasts, Snacks, Lunches and
    Dinners 303
28. Slow Carb Breakfasts, Snacks, Lunches and Dinners 326
29. What to Drink 352

References and Further Sources of Information 359
Resources 361
Index 369

Acknowledgements

Many people have helped with this book. Special thanks go to Professor Kieran Clarke, Professor Michael Crawford, Professor Stephen Cunnane, Professor David Ludwig, Dr David Unwin, Dr Zoe Harcombe, Dr Malcolm Kendrick, Ivan Crowe, Geoffrey Woo, Sue Wood of Charlie's Friends, Dr Robert Verkerk and Meleni Aldridge at the Alliance for Natural Health International (ANH-Intl), Marika Sboros, Marian Kalamian, Travis Christofferson and Paul Davies for their guidance and research; the team at diabetes.co.uk for their help and Fiona McDonald Joyce, co-author of *The Low GL Diet Cookbook*, for her delicious recipes. Also thanks to our editor Philip Parr and Jillian Stewart at Piatkus, and to Matthew Ingram for the illustrations and animation at hybriddiet.co.uk. We would also like to thank all of the amazing researchers out there whose studies have helped define a whole new natural, safe and healthy approach to today's endemic diseases.

Guide to Abbreviations
and Measures

1 gram (g) = 1000 milligrams (mg) = 1,000,000 micrograms (mcg or μg). Most vitamins are measured in milligrams or micrograms. Vitamins A, D and E are also measured in International Units (iu) – a measurement designed to standardise the different forms of these vitamins, which have different potencies.

1mcg of retinol (mcg RE) = 3.3iu of vitamin A (RE = Retinol Equivalents)
1mcg RE of beta-carotene = 6mcg
100iu of vitamin D = 2.5mcg
100iu of vitamin E = 67mg
1 pound (lb) = 16 ounces (oz)
2.2lb = 1 kilogram (kg)
1 cup = 240ml, ½ cup = 120ml, ¼ cup = 60ml

In this book, for simplicity, we use 'calories' in place of kilocalories (kcal).

Introduction

We have a problem – a serious problem. It's making millions of us chronically ill, pushing up the number of preventable deaths and threatening to bankrupt the National Health Service. We're suffering from a form of internal 'global warming' – an insidious change in the body's metabolism that lies behind the worldwide epidemics of obesity, diabetes, cancer and Alzheimer's disease. How we have got here – and what we should do about it – are the topics of this book.

According to public health guidelines, obesity is a major cause of cancer, diabetes and Alzheimer's. But what causes obesity itself? Well, that's easy. Officially, it is the result of ingesting too many calories. So, the recommended solution is to eat fewer calories. And since fat has more calories than either carbohydrate or protein, the theory goes that we should all eat less fat. But it is painfully obvious that this remedy is not working. This is because the less you eat, the hungrier you feel. Furthermore, you feel exhausted, so you are less likely to do any exercise and burn the calories you *have* eaten.

This book presents two alternative approaches that work for very clear but different reasons. It also explains why the conventional, calorie-controlled, low fat, high carb approach is sure to fail. Part 1 covers the ketogenic diet, which is based on eating large amounts of fat and virtually no carbs. We call this the 'high fat' approach. Part 2 focuses on the low glycemic load (or low GL) diet, which is based on eating slow-release carbs in controlled amounts. We call this the 'slow carb' approach.

If you eat nothing at all, your body takes emergency action and starts to break down your fat deposits. That's fine for your muscles but not so good for your brain – your most energy-hungry organ – because it cannot convert fat into energy. Its preferred fuel is glucose, which is derived from carbs, but the body stores only enough glucose to keep the brain going for a few days. Evolution solved this problem by developing ketones, which are made from the body's newly released fat and can be used to fuel *both* the brain and the muscles. Babies run on ketones for the first six months of life, as do penguins for four months each winter. Following the ketogenic diet as an adult helps weight loss because eating large quantities of fat and almost no carbs fools the body into thinking it is starving, so it converts its fat reserves into ketones. Furthermore, research suggests that this amazing fuel may have additional health benefits – such as switching the right genes on and off.

Ketones, or their direct precursors, may also be eaten or supplemented. In Chapter 19 – 'Good Fats' – you will learn about MCT oils (found in coconuts) and 'exogenous' ketone supplements, which can instantly boost the body's supply of ketones to levels that are normally achieved only after two days of fasting. Chapter 26 – 'Biohacking Your Ketone/Glucose Balance' – explains the effects that different diets have on your body and how to experiment with them. An increased level of ketones in the blood is called 'ketosis', while switching over from running on glucose to running on ketones – which happens during fasting or when following a high fat/low carb diet – is called 'ketogenesis', because your body makes the fuel from your own reserves of fat.

On the other hand, if you eat the right kind of (slow release) carbs in the right amounts, spread throughout the day, you will give your body a steady supply of glucose, which it can then convert into energy. From this perspective, strictly speaking, you only 'need' fat for essential nutrients such as omega-3 and -6 and vitamin D.

Developing the Hybrid Diet

I (Patrick) have spent the last thirty years developing, testing and improving the slow carb approach, which I call low GL (glycemic load). I've written *The Low GL Diet Bible*, *The Low GL Cookbook* and many other books that explain how to balance your blood sugar for steady energy, easy weight loss and disease reversal by stopping the conversion of excess glucose into fat.

I (Jerome) have spent the last five years knee deep in the science, the research and the politics behind ketogenic, high fat/low carb diets, and have seen the extraordinary results they are achieving against diabetes, cancer and brain diseases – from Alzheimer's to epilepsy.

Together, we will explain why mainstream medicine and government guidelines to tackle the obesity epidemic have got it so spectacularly wrong by demonising fat and glorifying carbs. We will also show you how and why both approaches – high fat and slow carb – work in simple, practical ways. Finally, we will explain why *alternating* between the two diets does more for your health than relying on just one. This is because, while both approaches may be described as 'low carb', they have different benefits.

The slow carb approach is a great, relatively easy way to stay healthy. You don't need to cut out carbs, just eat the right ones, and it will help you to lose weight. By contrast, the ketogenic diet is more demanding because you will need to substantially reduce your consumption of carbs, but the benefits are profound because it switches on various natural 'clean-up' and repair processes called 'autophagy' (see Chapter 14). This is most beneficial if you are in a 'disease' state, but it is also rejuvenating if you are healthy. Moreover, it may have an anti-ageing effect.

If you have kick-started your repair mechanisms with the high fat diet, you have the option of switching to slow carbs for a while. On the other hand, if you have been running on slow carbs for a few months, you might benefit from a metabolic clean-up by adopting the ketogenic diet. However, before we get on to the diets themselves, we'd like to tell you how this rich and fruitful collaboration started for us.

High Fat/Low Carbs

Five years ago, I (Jerome) attended a lecture in the British Library that changed the way I thought about food and health for ever. Previously, my views were largely off-the-shelf hand-me-downs: eat fat sparingly and go easy on the eggs, otherwise your arteries will clog up with fatty deposits, making a heart attack much more likely. That afternoon, these beliefs were turned upside down.

The speaker – Kieran Clarke, Professor of Physiological Biochemistry at Oxford University – explained that something remarkable happens when you cut your carbohydrate intake to almost zero and increase your consumption of fat to compensate. It was like a fairy story in which the one room you cannot enter in the castle contains not horrors but a wonderful new set of tools. I learned that you can get all the fuel you need from ketones, that carbs contain nothing you really require, and that this previously hidden system comes with its own dashboard that allows you to make tweaks and adjustments to the way your system runs that can improve health and help you handle any number of chronic diseases. Exciting or what?

I had stumbled on a revolution that was already well under way and would soon challenge not only the common consensus about diet and health but some long-standing assumptions about the way the human body works. Now, five years on, the idea of staying healthy by cutting down on carbs is fast becoming the new orthodoxy. Indeed, it has the potential to spark a medical revolution in the way we treat chronic disease.

The orthodox low fat regime was part of a medical approach that regarded the major chronic diseases as quite separate from one another. Heart disease was due to too much fat and cholesterol in the diet, which led to blocked arteries. Diabetes was the result of putting on too much weight, so the 'solution' was to cut consumption of calorie-dense fat. Cancer was due to random genetic mutations that caused the body's cells to go haywire, rather than the food we ate. Indeed, mainstream medical opinion encouraged patients to guzzle carbs in the form of cakes, puddings and ice cream so they had sufficient energy to tackle the disease. Alzheimer's was caused by damaged proteins killing off brain cells, a degenerative process that eventually decimated the patient's memory and cognitive functions. The standard advice was to reduce fat intake to keep the weight down, protect the heart and avoid diabetes, but eat plenty of carbohydrates for energy.

Traditionally, dietitians have played only a minor role in the treatment of any of these conditions. By contrast, the low carb movement – which encompasses advocates of both high fat and slow carb diets – places dietitians and nutritionists in the front line. It believes that they should work alongside doctors to help us overcome all of these diseases. This is not an eccentric, partisan view. Indeed, it is on the verge of becoming mainstream. For instance, it was one of the big ideas to emerge during a remarkable conference on nutrition organised by Swiss Re – one of the world's largest re-insurance companies – in Zurich in June 2018. Swiss Re is understandably alarmed by the rise of obesity and diabetes around the world, and it has reached the conclusion that low carbs, rather than low fat, is the best way to tackle the problem, keep its customers healthy for longer, and therefore reduce its pay-outs and increase its profits. The company's Chief Medical

Officer, Dr John Schoonbee, describes the last half-century's low fat approach as a 'failed human experiment'.

The highly respected *British Medical Journal*, one of the co-hosts of the Zurich conference, published a sixty-eight-page special edition on nutrition to coincide with the event. In her closing address to the conference, the editor, Dr Fiona Godlee, demanded a 'reversal' in the 'demonisation of fat' and issued a rallying call for the medical establishment to get up to speed with nutrition. 'Few areas of health are more important and more neglected in medical education,' she said, before expressing the hope that recent research into reversing diabetes and obesity through low carb diets might prove a 'tipping point'.

Indeed, the low carb approach has already been widely adopted in the treatment of diabetes. It's easy to see why this has happened: diabetics find it difficult to process glucose – the fuel that comes from carbohydrate-rich foods, such as bananas, bread and potatoes – so reducing their intake of carbs makes a lot of sense. Of course, this approach is also far cheaper than treating the condition with drugs.

Far more radical, however, is the idea that excessive glucose is not just related to diabetes. Cutting-edge research suggests that it might also be an early warning signal for the development of metabolic syndrome – an umbrella term for a cluster of symptoms including excess fat around the waist, increased blood pressure, high levels of fat (triglycerides) and inflammation. In turn, all of these are risk factors for developing one of the major chronic diseases – heart disease, cancer, Alzheimer's – so there are enormous benefits from tackling them before they take hold. Part 1 is all about how and why the high fat diet can help us achieve this.

Unfortunately, though, while the benefits of the ketogenic diet are undeniable, some people have taken this as their cue to demonise *all* carbohydrates and suggest that they are either unnecessary or even toxic. This is just as untrue and misleading as the opposite point of view. High fat and ketone research has revealed that humans are designed to use and switch between *two* types of fuel – ketones *and* glucose.

Our ancestors would have died out at the first sign of a famine if they had not developed the ability to use stored fat to power their muscles and brains when carbs were unavailable. We can store only about half a kilo of glucose – in the form of glycogen (one part glucose to four parts water) – in our muscles and liver, which is enough to keep us going for two or three days. That's why not eating for more than a couple of days triggers the liver to start making ketones from fat. These are small packets of energy which, crucially, can fuel the brain, since fat can't power the brain directly. Even if you are relatively lean, your fat deposits can be used by your muscles and metabolism, keeping you going for weeks. However, many of us now have no reason to access ketones as an energy source. The dependable food supply we have enjoyed in the West over the last sixty years has allowed us – and nutritional scientists – to believe that we can run continuously, and indefinitely, on nothing but carbohydrates. But living our whole lives without ever switching to ketones is like insisting on running a hybrid car only on petrol and refusing to use the batteries. Both of the car's power sources have their advantages and both should be used in certain circumstances, and it's exactly the same with the human body's use of carbs and ketones. The key to health is knowing what each one does and learning how to switch seamlessly between the two.

Slow Carbs

Meanwhile, I (Patrick) have been writing, teaching and helping people lose weight and reverse diseases with the slow carb/low GL diet for over twenty years. As with the high fat approach, fewer carbs are eaten to reduce the amount of glucose and hence insulin in the bloodstream, but the aim is not to push the body into ketosis.

Back in the 1990s, having established the Institute for Optimum Nutrition in 1984, I explored, researched and wrote about what constitutes 'optimum nutrition'. I concluded that weight control and diabetes prevention were all about stabilising blood sugar levels. My approach involved eating fewer carbs overall, and switching to foods with a low glycemic index (GI) and a low glycemic load (low GL): what we call 'slow carbs'. This meant that refined foods and sugar were out, but most other foods – eaten in the right quantities and combinations – were in. It's also entirely feasible for vegetarians and vegans. As you will see in Part 2, this method has achieved impressive results in reversing diabetes and heart disease, helping weight loss and even counteracting cancer and Alzheimer's.

If you eat low GL meals made up of slow carbs, your glucose level never climbs too high, nor do you trigger the flood of insulin that turns excess glucose into fat. There's also no big rebound glucose drop, so you are not left feeling hungry and tired after a meal. Therefore, eating slow carbs results in better weight control (or weight loss, if you need it), less hunger and more energy.

As I've seen thousands of clients achieve excellent results over the years, I must admit I've been rather sceptical about the 'need' to go to the extreme of eliminating almost all carbs in order to trigger ketosis. Why remove a whole food group that I (and millions of others) enjoy: wholegrain pasta, bread, cereals, potatoes, even root vegetables? For all its obvious virtues, is the ketogenic diet *really* the best way to lose weight and gain the associated health benefits? What about simply optimising your glucose engine, rather than switching to ketones? After all, it can take four days to push your body into ketosis, but only four minutes to get back to running on glucose.

However, as you will see later in this book, there are plenty of persuasive reasons to follow the ketogenic diet. In addition to being useful for weight loss, it can aid recovery from cancer, epilepsy and dementia. Furthermore, people who are heavily addicted to carbs often find it easier to avoid them completely by going down the ketogenic route rather than trying to cut down. Others choose this diet because they love meat and dairy products (although our high fat approach advises against making these foods staples). Most of all, though, there is convincing evidence that we should switch periodically between slow carbs and high fat, as we explain in Part 3.

I never bought into the low fat mantra, because I felt that the anti-fat science never stacked up. Instead, I have always recommended eggs and encouraged the consumption of healthy fats. This sounds like common sense today, but it was heresy twenty years ago. Indeed, I was hissed and booed on a late-night TV chat show for suggesting that sugar, not fat, was driving an obesity epidemic. The global healthcare cost of obesity is now estimated at over $2 trillion a year.

However, I was equally never convinced that grains – which supply more than half of the world's energy requirements and half of its protein – were the devil in disguise. The first civilisations thrived because of their cultivation of grain, and I saw no compelling reason to return to a hunter–gatherer existence, as some 'paleo' dieters suggest we should.

The old-school low fat, high carb, calorie-controlled diet – which was based on the idea that calories in (food) minus calories out (exercise) determines your weight – ignored the vast complexity of what happens in the interim, and it has proved utterly ineffectual at halting the global rise in obesity. Both a high fat and a slow carb approach work *with* your body's metabolism, increasing the calories you burn and reducing hunger; by contrast, low fat diets fight *against* your body, making you not only hungry but slothful and tired.[1]

We will suggest when a high fat approach is likely to be the better option, and when you should switch to slow carbs.

Eventually, though, you will become a master of your own metabolism, moving effortlessly between the two approaches. As a result, you will be able to eat more of your favourite foods more of the time. To help with this, measuring your glucose level will become as routine as checking your blood pressure and cholesterol levels. As an experiment, I recorded my blood glucose and ketone levels while writing this book. The former can be done with a meter that is strapped to the arm; the latter with a breathalyser that shows whether you are in ketosis (and therefore burning fat). In Part 4, we explain which foods pushed up blood glucose, and which raised the body's ketone level. You may be surprised by the results.

Three-quarters of the Hybrid Diet is identical whether you are in the slow carbs or the high fat phase: half of your total consumption is always vegetables and a little fruit, while a quarter is good-quality protein. The remaining quarter is *either* slow carbs *or* good fats. But don't concern yourself with the details just yet. After introducing the high fat/ketogenic diet in Part 1 and the slow carbs/low GL diet in Part 2, we will explain the benefits of alternating between the two in Part 3, tell you precisely how to combine them in Part 4, then present dozens of delicious recipes and mouth-watering menus in Part 5.

The path to health and wellbeing never tasted so good.

Part 1

Fat for Fuel

The low carb, high fat diet is the most exciting and radical development in dietary science over recent decades. It challenges the demonisation of fat, turns food consumption into an effective therapeutic tool and has the potential to revolutionise prevention and treatment of the world's major chronic diseases.

Chapter 1

The High Fat Ketone Revolution

Several years ago, a personal trainer called Sam Feltham subjected his body to a radical experiment. For three weeks, he ate identical low fat, high carb meals totalling a massive 5,000 calories each day (3,000 calories more than the recommended daily intake). Then, for the next three weeks, he continued to eat 5,000 calories a day, but this time all of his meals were high fat and low carbs. The aim of the experiment was to test two assumptions on which all official dietary advice was based.

The first of these assumptions was that the only way to lose weight is to eat fewer calories than you need to keep your metabolism going while increasing the amount you use by exercising. The second was that calorific value is all important: it's irrelevant whether the calories are contained in fat or carbohydrates.

Sam did a great deal of exercise, but even he assumed that he would pile on the pounds, given the amount he was eating over the course of the six weeks. Moreover, if the official guidance were correct, he should have put on exactly the same amount during the second three weeks as he did in the first part of the experiment. It did not turn out that way, though. As expected, on the low fat, high carb diet, Sam stacked on 16lb and gained 3.7in (9.5cm) around his middle. However, he added just 2½lb and *lost* 1in (3cm) from his waistline in phase two.

This result may have confounded many a dedicated weight-watcher, with years of skimmed milk and margarine under their belts, but it merely confirmed what Feltham himself had long suspected. He was a member of a group of nutrition radicals – journalists, academics, clinicians and a handful doctors – who had started to challenge the prevailing public health mantra that all fat – and especially saturated fat – was the root of all dietary evil.

This notion was the brainchild of an American physiologist named Ancel Keys, who from the 1950s onwards almost single-handedly persuaded politicians and doctors to accept his ideas on the basis of specious research. In the process, he ruthlessly disparaged the work of an eminent contemporary, the British professor John Yudkin, who believed that sugar was the real culprit. Now, thankfully, Keys's star has waned and a new generation of researchers, including US academics Gerald Reaven and Jeff Volek, are following in Yudkin's footsteps. Their studies suggest that insulin, which clears excess glucose from the blood, plays a role in the development of heart disease and other chronic illnesses. Moreover, they believe that, as a high carb diet results in regular, inevitable increases in blood glucose, the body gradually becomes desensitised to insulin – a condition known as insulin resistance. The key to preventing or reversing this condition is to eat fewer carbs.

One of the pre-eminent nutrition radicals is US journalist Nina Teicholz, who became her newspaper's restaurant critic and 'found myself eating things that had hardly ever passed my lips before: pâté, beef, cream sauces. To my surprise, I lost ten pounds that I hadn't been able to shake for years, and my cholesterol levels improved to boot.' Teicholz spent the next ten years interviewing America's leading dietary experts and then writing a remarkably detailed – but very readable – book titled *Big Fat Surprise*. 'I was shocked to find egregious flaws in the science that has served as the foundation for our national nutrition policy,' she says, 'a policy that has all but forbidden these delicious – *and healthy* – foods for fifty years.'

Among a host of startling discoveries, Teicholz learned that the committee responsible for compiling 'Dietary Guidelines for Americans', which had advocated the low fat diet for decades, had routinely ignored all scientific evidence to the contrary (of which there was plenty). She also refuted Keys's claim that the inhabitants of Crete had a low rate of heart disease because they ate an almost fat-free diet. It turned out that he had conducted his interviews during Lent, when the Cretans ate no meat, fish, eggs, cheese or butter. But they happily consumed all of these foods throughout the rest of the year. By contrast, they ate – and continue to eat – almost no refined sugar.

Another radical, Dr Zoe Harcombe, studied a 1977 US Senate Committee report that pinned all of the blame for America's heart disease epidemic on fat. She found that the report relied on just six relatively small-scale experiments, all of which were conducted 'in the absence of supporting evidence from randomised controlled trials (RCTs)' – an inexcusable oversight in any medical research.[1] Next, Harcombe analysed twenty subsequent experiments (involving a total of 60,000 people) that *did* incorporate RCTs: 2.16 per cent of the participants who were placed on a low fat diet suffered a heart attack, compared with only 1.80 per cent of those in the control groups. The overall conclusion was that while the low fat diet significantly lowered cholesterol, this had no obvious health benefits.[2] If anything, as Harcombe's analysis revealed, it seemed to have a detrimental impact on heart health.

This finding backed up an earlier meta-analysis of 72 studies involving more than 600,000 participants across 18 countries, which suggested that people who ate saturated fat were no more likely to develop heart disease than those who filled their trolleys with low fat yoghurts and skinless chicken. It also found that boosting your intake of supposedly 'healthy' fats, such as olive oil and corn oil, provided no more protection than tucking into the universally condemned rib-eye steak and butter. The conclusion was stark: 'Saturated fats do not cause heart disease.' Yet, it seemed that even the authors could not quite believe their findings, because they merely offered the tentative suggestion that 'more large-scale clinical studies are needed'.[3] This provided a get-out clause for the public health authorities: they refused to act on the evidence that was already staring them in the face and continued to proclaim the supposed benefits of the low fat diet.

Harcombe has now turned her attention to the theory that you will lose weight as long as you use more energy than you consume in food. 'It's important to dispel this particular myth because it is one of the crutches that are used to support the demonisation of fat,' she says. 'Fat contains twice as many calories as carbohydrates, so if calories have the same effect wherever they come from, you should avoid fat if you want to lose weight.' A pound of fat contains about 3,500 calories and you might ingest 500 fewer calories on a regular weight-loss diet each day, so losing a pound of fat should take around seven days. 'You usually lose more to begin with and less later,' explains Harcombe, 'but the calculation still suggests that you will be twenty-one to twenty-six pounds lighter after six months. But that *never* happens in studies or clinical experience. Instead, the normal result is that you lose around ten pounds after six months, then put it all back on over the next six months, even though – and this is the important point – you are still eating five hundred fewer calories each day.'

If the 'calories in/calories out' equation is flawed, that creates serious problems for the whole low fat approach. First, it suggests that different macro-nutrients do indeed have different effects on the body – as supporters of the high fat, low carb diet claim. When you eat carbohydrates, they are turned into glucose and released into the bloodstream, so your blood glucose level rises. This is followed by an automatic release of insulin, which converts excess glucose into fat in the liver. The fat is then delivered to the body's fat cells for storage. As long as the fat stores are replenished from surplus glucose, the system doesn't allow any fat to be released. However, if carbohydrate supplies start to decrease – as they do on a high fat diet – both blood glucose and insulin levels decline, too. At that point, the body's automatic response is to release fat from its reserves. Consequently, you start to lose weight. However, while most of the body's cells can use the fat itself, rather than glucose, as their energy source, brain cells cannot. Fortunately, the liver solves this problem by converting some of the newly released fat into ketones – energy-dense molecules that the brain and the muscles can use as a sort of high octane fuel.

Armed with this knowledge, the conclusion is obvious: a diet that is high in carbohydrates will continuously top up your blood glucose, which your body will continuously convert into fat. By contrast, you will not put on weight if you eat a high fat diet because your blood glucose level drops and there is no surplus to turn into body fat. The idea of simply eating fewer carbs and exercising more to lose the pounds is a sweet fallacy. The crucial factor is *what* you eat.

Nevertheless, Western governments, dietitians and public health bodies were all hoodwinked by the fallacy, especially after the US Senate Committee published its deeply flawed report in 1977. This was great news for the sugar industry. Fizzy drinks and confectionery companies enthusiastically supported the officially approved low fat diet and, to drive the message home, sponsored major sporting events at which they were able to promote the supposed health benefits of their products. Of course, in reality, these companies were far more interested in promoting their brands and increasing their profits.

Coca-Cola was one of these highly visible corporate sponsors, but it also employed somewhat more dubious tactics to promote the alleged benefits of the low fat diet according to an investigative article in the BMJ published in April 2018.[4] For instance, the company donated $1.5 million to a non-profit organisation called Global Energy Balance Network (GEBN), as well as many millions more to fund the research of academics who were connected to the organisation. GEBN was finally wound up in 2015, but by then it had sponsored dozens of clinical trials, all of which – surprise, surprise – seemed to prove the efficacy of the low-fat approach.

The organisation presented itself as an 'honest broker' that aimed to 'reframe the discussion' on the causes of obesity in the Western world. In reality, its role was to promote the interests of Coca-Cola and the other major corporate players in the 'growing war between the public health community and private industry about how to reduce obesity'. Coca-Cola was especially concerned about plans to 'tax or ban foods that are considered unhealthy', which one of the company's executives described as 'extreme solutions' to the obesity problem. However, she admitted that the corporation's intention was to 'promote best practices that are effective in terms of both policy *and profit* (emphasis added)'.[5] Even by US corporate standards, this attempt to increase Coke's profits by funding a supposedly impartial research organisation was particularly cynical.

On the other hand, on occasion, major corporations' overriding concern with the bottom line can be beneficial. For instance, in a 2015 report, the global banking giant Credit Suisse found that high fat foods are a safe and effective means of preventing and treating obesity, diabetes and heart disease. Therefore, the report concluded that such foods will inevitably increase in popularity, which 'offers powerful investment ideas'.[6] Similarly, as we saw in the Introduction (see page xix), insurance companies, such as Swiss Re, have a vested interest in keeping their clients alive and healthy for as long as possible; as a result, they are also advocating the high fat diet.

The Fat Cholesterol Con

Perhaps the most trenchant critique of the low fat approach comes from Dr Malcolm Kendrick, a British GP and author of *The Great Cholesterol Con*. He argues that low fat diets simply don't make sense, because no fat – saturated or otherwise – has a direct effect on cholesterol level.[7] 'This is basic physiology,' he says. 'Each of them [fat and cholesterol] is carried round the body in a different transport system. They don't interact.'

After we eat fat, it arrives in the gut, where it is packed into very large containers known as chylomicrons and delivered directly into the bloodstream. Crucially, these containers do not head for the liver at this point. Rather, they take most of their cargo straight to fat stores and shrink as they deposit their loads. Only then do they proceed to the liver for recycling. By contrast, cholesterol is made in the liver and then packed into containers called VLDLs (very low-density lipoproteins) along with fat (triglycerides). These containers then travel through the bloodstream, shrinking as they deliver their cargo. When they are almost empty – and now known as LDLs – they return to the liver for recycling.

If so-called 'bad' LDL cholesterol comes from VLDLs, the key question is: what increases the number of VLDLs in the bloodstream? It can't be fat because that is transported in chylomicrons, rather than VLDLs. The answer is carbohydrates!

If you eat more carbs than your body can use or store, the liver converts the excess into saturated fat, packs it into VLDLs and launches it into the bloodstream. So, if you eat fat, your VLDL level falls. If you eat carbohydrates, your VLDL level rises.[8]

The theory is utterly convincing and supported by highly positive results among diabetics who have reversed their condition by adopting high fat diets. Yet, public health bodies and dietitians have stubbornly refused to abandon the low fat approach. Indeed, some professional bodies' response has been closer to a witch hunt than an objective consideration of the evidence. For instance, in Australia in 2016, the Australian Health Practitioners' Regulatory Authority launched an investigation into the work of Dr Gary Fettke, an orthopaedic surgeon with twenty-three years' experience.[9] This followed an anonymous complaint from a dietitian that Fettke was unqualified to give nutritional advice after he had urged several diabetic patients to try a high fat diet or risk losing one or both of their feet – a consequence of diabetes. Amazingly, the subsequent hearing ordered Fettke to stop dispensing nutritional advice, and specifically to stop advising his patients to give up sugar. Even more remarkably, it insisted that he must continue to keep his counsel on nutritional matters if – or when – official guidelines changed in the future, regardless of whether these accepted that Fettke was right all along. In September 2018 all charges were dropped.

It should be pointed out that this wasn't an isolated case of a doctor who was reprimanded for offering advice outside of his area of expertise. Around the same time, a New South Wales dietitian, Jennifer Elliott, was expelled from the Dietitians Association of Australia for recommending the low carb diet to patients with type 2 diabetes. The association then issued a stern warning to its remaining members that 'nutritional advice to clients must not include a low carbohydrate diet'. Elliott's response was incredulous: 'Can you imagine having to tell a client with diabetes, who has lowered his blood glucose levels, lost weight and come off all diabetes medications by reducing his carb intake, that he now has to start eating more carbs because SNSW Health says so?'[10]

Meanwhile, in South Africa, a battle over LCHF between senior scientist and specialist in sports nutrition Professor Tim Noakes and the Health Professions Council of South Africa (HPCSA) was well underway. The council had charged Noakes (who had recently come out in favour of the high fat diet on the grounds it was more physiologically plausible) with unprofessional conduct for giving 'unconventional advice to a breastfeeding mother on a social network'. The mother had asked: 'Is LCHF eating OK for breastfeeding mums? Worried about all the dairy + cauliflower = wind for babies?? [sic]' Noakes had responded: 'Baby doesn't eat the dairy and cauliflower. Just very healthy high fat breast milk. Key is to ween [sic] baby onto LCHF.' Since the LCHF diet includes meat, fish, dairy and vegetables, there is nothing here that conflicted with conventional advice.

The official grounds for the hearing included that he was providing a medical consultation online and that his advice was unconventional. After a drawn-out legal hearing, Noakes was eventually found not guilty of all charges in 2018. The mother was not his patient, his response did not constitute a consultation and LCHF was not unconventional. Like the Fettke case, it appeared to be a huge over-reaction, and possibly one that had more to do with protecting professional turf.

A couple of years earlier, Noakes had written a textbook on sports nutrition in which he had recommended the standard low fat diet, but he told the HPCSA that he had subsequently changed his mind and now found the high fat approach much more physiologically plausible. Yet, the council seemed uninterested in what had persuaded an eminent scientist with 500 peer-reviewed publications to his name and several life-time achievement awards to make such a radical shift. Instead, it simply charged him with 'unprofessional conduct' because he had provided 'unconventional advice on breastfeeding'.[11] Thankfully, though, after an extremely stressful three-year investigation, he was exonerated.

One of Noakes's star witnesses at his hearing was Nina Teicholz, who had recently highlighted 'weak methods' that did not reflect the 'best and most current science' in the latest version of the 'Dietary Guidelines for Americans'.[12] She says, 'After doing the book [*The Big Fat Surprise*], I couldn't understand how they yet again supported limiting saturated fats and failed to mention the benefits of low carb diets for those battling obesity. Looking at the report in detail, I found this was done by ignoring dozens of rigorous studies on low carb diets, [including] several long-term trials lasting two years which demonstrated that these diets are safe and highly effective for combating obesity, diabetes and heart disease.' Teicholz's conclusion is that officially recommended diets are generally based on a 'minuscule quantity of rigorous evidence that only marginally support claims that these diets can promote better health than alternatives'.

Unsurprisingly, the low fat lobby has not taken Teicholz's claims lying down. One group, the Center for Science in the Public Interest (CPSI), organised a petition that was signed by more than 170 researchers and academics, including every member of the committee that had drafted the latest 'Dietary Guidelines for Americans'. This called for a full retraction of the 2015 *British Medical Journal* article in which Teicholz had presented her arguments, on the basis that it contained eleven serious factual errors. The journal responded by commissioning an external review, which found that just a couple of minor points should be corrected. Otherwise, the *BMJ* was able to stand by all of Teicholz's findings and conclusions, so it refused to withdraw her article.

'Eatwell' Equals Eat Badly

The low fat lobby's demonisation of fat has been disastrous. It has allowed the true culprit in the obesity epidemic – sugar – to escape scrutiny, increased sugar intake, driven down consumption of essential omega-3 fats and vital vitamin D, duped countless dietitians and public health bodies, and twisted research to support its claims.

A prime example of this flawed thinking is the officially approved 'Eatwell Guide', which is seriously unbalanced. It says a healthy diet should be eaten in the proportions shown on the plate opposite: 37 per cent starchy carbs, 39 per cent fruit and

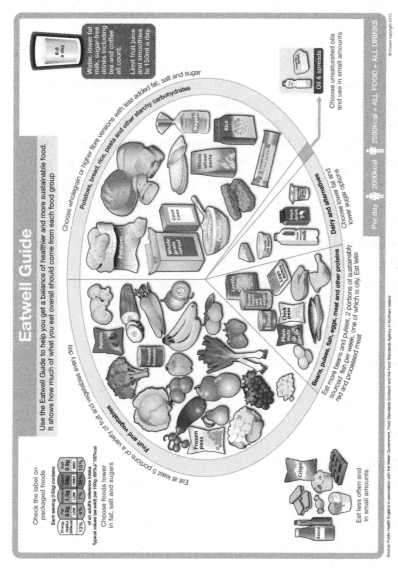

Eatwell Guide

Use the Eatwell Guide to help you get a balance of healthier and more sustainable food. It shows how much of what you eat overall should come from each food group.

Check the label on packaged foods

Each serving (150g) contains

Energy 1046kJ 250kcal	Fat 3.0g	Saturates 1.3g	Sugars 34g	Salt 0.9g
13%	4%	LOW 7%	HIGH 38%	MED 15%

of an adult's reference intake
Typical values (as sold) per 100g: 697kJ/167kcal

Choose foods lower in fat, salt and sugars

Eat at least 5 portions of a variety of fruit and vegetables every day

Fruit and vegetables

Potatoes, bread, rice, pasta and other starchy carbohydrates

Choose wholegrain or higher fibre versions with less added fat, salt and sugar

6-8 a day

Water, lower fat milk, sugar-free drinks including tea and coffee all count.

Limit fruit juice and smoothies to 150ml a day.

Oil & spreads

Choose unsaturated oils and use in small amounts

Dairy and alternatives

Choose lower fat and lower sugar options

Beans, pulses, fish, eggs, meat and other proteins

Eat more beans and pulses, 2 portions of sustainably sourced fish per week, one of which is oily. Eat less red and processed meat

Eat less often and in small amounts

Per day   2000kcal   2500kcal = ALL FOOD + ALL DRINKS

Source Public Health England in association with the Welsh Government, Food Standards Scotland and the Foods Standards Agency in Northern Ireland vegetables, 8 per cent dairy and 12 per cent beans, pulses, fish, eggs and meat. What it doesn't tell you is how many calories you'll get from each section.

When Dr Zoe Harcombe did that calculation a very different picture of what we 'should' be eating emerged.[13] Calories from starchy carbs would make up 60 per cent or a whopping 71 per cent (375 grams) if you added in foods from a section described as 'eat sparingly and less often'; in other words cakes, sweets and fizzy drinks – all junk carbohydrates. They make up 9 per cent your daily calories. Astonishingly, fruit and vegetables now only make up 6 per cent of total calories.

The odd category that combines beans, pulses, meat, fish and eggs – some of the most nutritious foods – supplies only 10 to 12 per cent of total calories. 'Eating to get the proportions of your daily calories from this guide,' says Dr Harcombe 'means that you will be getting insufficient fat/protein and excess carbohydrate. You will be under nourished nutritionally and over-fed fuel.'

In addition, your intake of omega-3 fats – which are found mainly in oily fish, nuts and seeds – would be a fraction of the optimal levels required for good health.

So, it turns out that the supposedly healthy, balanced low fat diet is unhealthy and seriously unbalanced.[14] Bin it.

Chapter 2

High Fat, Low Carb
Reverses Diabetes

Diabetes is one of our biggest and most expensive health problems, and there is a desperate need for a more effective treatment. Currently, around 3.2 million people in the United Kingdom have been diagnosed with type 2 diabetes, but this figure is increasing by 5 per cent every year. The direct cost to the NHS is nearly £10 billion – 10 per cent of its total budget. Worldwide, diabetes affects 422 million people and costs over $825 billion, with 90 per cent of cases type 2.

The UK first issued guidelines recommending a low fat, high carb diet in 1983. Since then, millions have followed the official advice, yet diabetes and obesity have increased exponentially. With the benefit of hindsight, this was inevitable because the government was trying to treat a disorder involving excessive levels of sugar and insulin with a diet that causes both to rise several times each day. Drugs have been developed to combat the disease, but these are mostly designed to allow patients to continue to eat a high carb diet by reducing blood sugar levels pharmacologically. If you like cake, the usual advice is to increase your dose to compensate!

Surely, it would be a better idea simply to reduce your intake of carbohydrates, which would result in an automatic reduction in your insulin level – a driver of many of the key symptoms of diabetes, including weight gain, insulin resistance and chronic inflammation. Understandably, this approach makes a lot of sense to diabetics themselves, and it is recommended on the website www.diabetes.co.uk (not to be confused with the official charity Diabetes UK, which is at www.diabetes.org.uk).

This site was a revelation to Dr David Unwin, a GP from Lancashire. He was amazed to read the testimonies of patients who were enthusiastic about the high fat diet and reported some astonishing results: 5–6kg lost in a few months; glucose and insulin levels right down; no need for drugs. 'To be honest,' Unwin says, 'I had begun to despair of being able to do much for my patients with diabetes. Most found it very hard to lose weight, so I'd start by warning patients that if they didn't control their blood sugar and weight with diet, they would have to go on drugs. But nutrition was never my field, so I'd send them to the dietitian, who would advise a low fat, high carb diet.'

Inevitably, this approach almost always failed, so Unwin looked for an alternative and advised nineteen of his patients to follow the low carb, high fat diet he had seen on the diabetes website. This entailed drastic reductions in their consumption of starchy bread, rice and pasta as well as sugary products. By the end of the eight-month trial, only two of the patients still had high glucose levels, but even these had declined substantially. The participants lost an average of 9kg, their blood pressure was lower, and they experienced significant improvements in their levels of gamma-glutamyl transferase (GGT), an important indicator of liver health.[15]

Diabetes UK responded to Unwin's findings, which he published in 2014, by declaring that there was insufficient evidence for the 'long-term safety' of the diet. As such, it ignored the fact that the National Institute for Health and Care Excellence (NICE) recommends a version of the low carb diet for children with severe epilepsy, which they are advised to follow for years (see Chapter 6).

Next, Unwin turned his attention to the two different types of carbohydrate – those that raise blood sugar rapidly (high GL) and those that release their sugar gradually (low GL). He advised diabetics to consume only low GL carbohydrates and saw 'significant improvements in diabetes control and weight, while spending around £40,000 less per year on diabetes drugs'.[16]

Such findings have 'totally changed the way we run the surgery,' says Unwin. 'Now I collaborate with diabetic patients on their problems with weight. I ask them about their goals and what they hope to achieve. If I get involved with what they are doing, they often surprise me with the changes they are prepared to make.' By 2017, his practice had cut its drugs bill by £50,000 a year, and over 200 of his fellow GPs had joined an online low carb group to share advice and findings.

The Ketogenesis Pioneers

While David Unwin advocated the careful control of carbohydrates, plenty of diabetic patients and a few clinicians were prepared to go much further by reducing their carb intake to as little as 20g a day, while increasing their consumption of fat. In short, they adopted a full-blown ketogenic diet and forced their bodies into ketogenesis. There was no more calorie counting, but they had to abandon all of the low-fat staples, including skimmed milk, ready meals with added sugar, and starchy foods, such as bread and potatoes. These foodstuffs were replaced with plenty of meat, poultry, fish, eggs and full-fat cheese, along with unlimited amounts of cream, avocado, coconut oil, seeds, nuts and olives (and their oils).

As we explained in the Introduction, ketogenesis is the body's natural response to starvation. Once the body has exhausted its limited reserves of glucose, it first converts protein from our muscles into glucose, which is used to fuel the brain. However, this is not a good long-term solution, given that we need our muscles as well as our brain, so the body soon switches to the production of ketones. These are made from fat that is released from storage in response to the critical carbohydrate shortage, and they are a perfect source of energy for both the brain and the muscles. The body still needs a small amount of glucose on a daily basis, but this can be manufactured from protein. That's why it's important to eat plenty of protein if you are on a high fat diet.

Inducing ketogenesis through starvation is a fairly unpleasant process, and obviously it cannot be sustained for very long. By contrast, the ketogenic diet is a way of achieving precisely the same effect without the pain and for an indefinite period of time. Lowering (or eliminating) the carbs causes the shift while the extra fat in the diet stops the hunger.

Adopting this approach certainly helped John, a sixty-six-year-old type 2 diabetic from Bristol. He was informed that he would have to start on medication unless he reduced his weight significantly within the next three months. This alarmed him, not least because he was already taking pills following a heart attack. However, previous attempts at weight loss had all failed, and he had no idea what to try next. 'My doctor just said eat smaller portions, but that hadn't helped. And the diabetic nurse weighed at least eighteen stone, so I didn't take her advice very seriously.' Then John stumbled across the diabetes.co.uk website. 'It was a godsend,' he says. 'Their low carb programme took ten weeks and came with lots of comments and support from other diabetics who were raving about the amount of weight they'd lost.'

John and his wife Di decided to undertake the programme together, despite a degree of initial apprehension. 'It was scary to begin with,' says Di. 'All that meat, extra fat – butter and full-fat milk – foods we'd been warned to avoid for years. Staying off carbohydrates when they are everywhere was tricky, too.' John lost 2 stone (13kg) and didn't need to go on the threatened medication, while Di lost 5.5kg. 'I think bread and potatoes were our downfall. We've cut them right out,' she says.

Overall, participants in the diabetes.co.uk programme report an average weight loss of 7.4kg and an average reduction in the key blood sugar marker – HbA1c – of 1.2 per cent. (By contrast, diabetics on the standard low fat diet usually gain weight and see increases in their levels of HbA1c.) Even more striking is that 39 per cent have lowered their HbA1c to a point where they are no longer considered diabetic, while 40 per cent have been able to stop taking one or more drugs for the condition. It has been estimated that the NHS saves £814.36 per year for every patient who comes off diabetes medication. Many of the participants also report alleviation of some of the classic symptoms of diabetes, such as insomnia and lack of energy.

Nevertheless, Britain's health authorities have refused to take these findings seriously, dismissing the thousands of testimonials as anecdotal. In response, Arjun Panasar, the founder of diabetes. co.uk, argues, 'It's very short-sighted to ignore big data. It's potentially far more flexible and informative than large, cumbersome and very expensive randomised trials. When you have information on what people are eating, what drugs they are taking, how much sleep and exercise they are getting, you can match it with changes in their weight, blood sugar levels and symptoms. Do that on 10,000 people and you start to know what works. Big data plus patient involvement is the medicine of the future.'

Overcoming Resistance

The low carb diet also seems to be highly effective in combating insulin resistance – a serious condition that is associated with pre-diabetes as well as diabetes itself. The effect is similar to addiction – your body needs ever more insulin to get the same effect as cells become less and less responsive to the hormone. As a result, weight, blood pressure and blood glucose all increase. The pancreas reacts by secreting even more insulin, which has damaging effects throughout the body. In response, the insulin-resistant fat cells start to send out inflammatory chemical messengers (cytokines), which inflame the cells' mitochondrial power plants. The end results are chronic tiredness and accelerated ageing. However, a number of recent scientific studies have found that a high fat diet can help to arrest or even reverse this process.[17]

The largest and most impressive of these trials involved 262 diabetic patients who were restricted to 30g of carbs a day for two years. Meanwhile, most of their energy needs were met by an increased intake of fat. At the start of the study, the average HbA1c level (a marker of how high their blood glucose had been recently) was 7.6 per cent, but after ten weeks 50 per cent had a level of 6.5 per cent, meaning they were technically in remission. Similarly, at the beginning of the trial, nine out of ten participants were taking at least one drug; by the end, more than half had either reduced or ceased their medication altogether.[18] Moreover, they probably felt far more content throughout the two-year experiment, because another study reported a 'significant decrease in the psychological stress associated with diabetes management alongside a reduction in negative moods between meals'.[19]

Low Cal or High Fat?

So, the evidence against high carbs and in favour of high fat is mounting all the time, and thousands of diabetics have already benefited as a result. However, scientists are always searching for the next big thing, and one group of researchers recently trialled a drastic approach that limited 300 participants to just 800 calories in the form of a liquid nutritional supplement each day. On average, the patients lost 10kg over the course of the year-long experiment and nearly half managed to reverse their diabetes.[20] Anyone who knew anything about diet and diabetes could have predicted this result. After all, the participants effectively starved themselves to initiate ketogenesis. But is this approach really preferable to the much more straightforward high fat diet, which achieves equally impressive results, as we have seen? As Zoe Harcombe says, 'What would you prefer? A very low *calorie* diet, which comes with hunger, nutritional deficiency, inability to socialise and lifelong demands on your willpower? Or low *carbohydrate*, which avoids hunger, is nutritionally rich, is catered for in any restaurant – from McDonald's (no bun) to The Ivy – and can be sustained without monk-like discipline?'

It briefly seemed as though the liquid diet might have something new to offer, as a follow-up study found that those participants who went into remission experienced 'sustained improvement' in their insulin-producing beta-cells.[21] However, around the same time, another group of researchers reported that a ketogenic diet achieved precisely the same result without any need for draconian, long-term calorie restriction.[22] True, their study involved mice, rather than humans, but the animals were put on a 'fasting mimicking diet', which is already used in the treatment of human diabetes. This is basically a high fat diet in which the calorific intake is cut in half, but only for five days each month. More research is needed, but the early results are interesting.

However, is there really any need to look for alternatives to

David Unwin's tried and tested approach? As he says, 'Be relaxed about quantities, aim to eat a variety of good, fresh food, and be sparing with refined food. Good bread or roast potatoes are fine occasionally, although if you are diabetic you'll do better to avoid such foods until your blood sugar is under control. And eat at least enough fat to make your food tasty.' Since he started recommending the low carb, high fat diet, 46 per cent of Unwin's diabetes patients have achieved drug-free partial remission.

But that leaves one final question: what do we mean by low carbs? To some extent, the figure varies from person to person, and you will need to find a level that suits you (see Chapter 26 for more details). However, if you follow official, government-approved dietary advice, you will eat about 225g of carbohydrate each day. As a first step to going low carb, you should aim to reduce this to about 130g, and then to 50g after a couple of weeks. A further reduction to 20–30g will take you into ketogenic territory. We explore all of this – including the advantages of low GL carbs – in much more detail in Parts 2 and 4.

Chapter 3

The High Fat Cancer Hope

A low carb diet for diabetes makes sense because it rapidly reduces the amount of glucose and insulin in the blood, and diabetics have a problem with controlling both. The link with cancer is not so obvious because cancer is supposedly the result of rogue gene mutations. However, PET body scans that tell you where your cancer is, also reveal the glucose connection. That's because the way scanners identify cancer cells is by responding to massively increased glucose consumption. Cancer cells are voracious for sugar to fuel their rapid growth, so starving cancer seems a good strategy.

Raffi's Story

In 2007, Miriam Kalamian, an American business woman, scoured the internet for something that might help her seven-year-old son Raffi, who was suffering from seemingly terminal brain cancer. She came across an article by Dr Thomas Seyfried, a researcher at Boston University who reported that he had slowed down or even reversed the growth of tumours in lab animals by feeding them a high fat, ketogenic diet. This involved drastically reducing the animals' intake of carbohydrates, which reduced their level of blood glucose and soon pushed them into ketosis. Crucially, it seemed that those little packets of energy that are so valuable for the brain and the muscles – ketones – were use-less to the tumours. They needed glucose to grow ... and there wasn't any!

It was a very long shot, but Raffi had already undergone two unsuccessful operations and he was responding very badly to a new cocktail of chemotherapy. The tumour was still growing, putting increasing pressure on his brain. He was constantly nau-seous, fatigued and unable to focus. One morning, he collapsed and started talking gibberish. 'Raffi desperately needed some-thing different,' said Miriam. 'After all, what did we have to lose?'

Miriam was a pioneer when she put Raffi on a high fat diet. In effect, she set off alone with little in the way of guidance, back-up or advice from the oncology establishment. However, there was a ray of hope. Another group of clinicians had already prescribed high fat diets for children with severe epilepsy, and the results were remarkable, with 80 per cent of the patients experiencing a reduction in seizures. So, high fat diets had proved effective in the treatment of seriously ill children, but there was no hard evidence that it would have a similar impact on Raffi's brain cancer.

Indeed, many self-proclaimed experts soon issued dire warn-ings: Raffi would get insufficient nutrients from the new diet and his ketone levels would increase, which could kill him. Amazingly, though, within three months, Raffi's tumour had shrunk by 10 to 15 per cent. Meanwhile, his quality of life improved dramatically and he returned to the talkative, energetic little boy he had been before the illness. His remarkably open-minded oncologist had predicted that he had just a one-in-three chance of responding to the diet, and just a one-in-ten chance that any response would continue for eighteen months. In fact, he survived for another six years. 'Much of the time he was living pretty normally,' says Miriam. 'Even towards the end, we were riding bikes around town and swimming at our favourite hot springs.'

Nevertheless, more than a decade later, treating cancer with high fat diets is still considered beyond the medical pale. Indeed, the UK's largest cancer charity terms the approach a 'myth'. Yet, thousands have followed Miriam's lead, and there are now even some guides to help you on the journey. Miriam herself was so impressed by the results that she enrolled in a nutrition degree and has spent the last ten years dispensing information to others. Her detailed and compelling book – *Keto for Cancer* – was published in 2017.[23]

The official line of the cancer charities and the medical establishment is that there have been no rigorous scientific studies into the treatment of cancer with high fat diets. But this merely begs the question: *why* have there been no trials, especially as the approach's efficacy in the treatment of epilepsy has been well known for more than a century?[24] Belatedly, though, there are some signs that the high fat diet might be inching into the mainstream. For instance, several cautiously favourable pieces of research were published in the summer of 2017, including one which found that a common cancer drug was more effective when mice were put on the diet.[25] One of the drug's usual side-effects is raised blood glucose, but the high fat diet counteracted this and the tumours shrank as a result. Even the NHS has admitted that the approach is 'tolerable and feasible', and research among patients suggests that most would be willing to participate in trials.[26]

When Raffi started on the diet, a major obstacle was the official dietary advice, which stated that cancer patients should avoid fat and fill up on carbs instead. However, as we have seen, recent reports of the high fat diet's success in reversing diabetes should prompt a rethink about its use among cancer patients. This is because both disorders are linked to high levels of glucose and insulin in the bloodstream, and diabetes itself is a significant risk factor for cancer.

Then there are the individual success stories.

Charles's Story

One UK patient – let's call him Charles – developed a 'vascular highly malignant brain tumour', known as an anaplastic astrocytoma, in 2013. The chemotherapy left him feeling terrible, so he decided to abandon it and turned to the high fat diet instead. Young, fit and a personal trainer with a degree in sports nutrition, he felt it was worth the risk, although his oncologist warned him that the diet would have no effect on the tumour, and cutting out carbs would be dangerous because his brain needed glucose to function. Charles ignored the advice and began the standard ketogenic combination of reducing his intake of carbs and replacing the lost calories with low sugar fruits and vegetables, coconut milk and oil, nuts, cheese, avocados and so on. Unfortunately, this diet left him feeling 'absolutely awful': his migraines and seizures – common side effects of brain cancer – grew so bad that he remained in bed for months.

However, Charles didn't give up. Indeed, rather than going back to chemotherapy, he had the courage to try an even more high-risk strategy. Having searched through the internet, he learned that his symptoms might be due to a reaction to salicylates in the plant foodstuffs he was eating, so he cut all of them out immediately. 'The result was amazing,' he says. 'The headaches and seizures reduced almost at once.' But this left Charles with a major challenge: how could he replace what had become the staples of his diet? After further research, he concluded that he could meet all of his nutritional needs with animal-based foodstuffs.

Thereafter, Charles continued to tinker with his diet until he achieved the best possible balance for his personal needs. At first, he relied on bone broth and organ meats (liver, kidney, brain and sweetbreads), which kept his headaches and seizures at bay while his brain scans continued to show improvement. Then he took another leap: 'I added insects to my diet, along with some MCT [medium-chain triglyceride] oil, which the liver can turn directly into ketones [see Chapter 5]. I've tried other versions over the last few years, but this particular zero carb ketogenic diet is the only one that has given me near-complete symptom relief. The ingredients include two to four eggs, liver, lamb's brain from a local sheep farmer, sardines or mackerel, bone broth, crickets or other insects, such as wax worms, bacon or red meat with Cheddar cheese.'

Many people would find it impossible to follow such a diet: it comprises over 200g of fat and 70–75g of protein each day. Moreover, most nutritionists would probably consider it dangerous. But it works for Charles, and it illustrates just how flexible the ketogenic diet can be. And he is still experimenting. For instance, he recently introduced raw cacao, a form of MCT called C8 from coconut oil (see Chapter 19) and even home-grown sprouted broccoli (which is rich in an anti-seizure compound). He also fasts every few months (see Chapter 15).

The Oncologists' Response

The lack of scientific trials and the persistent assumption that cancer cannot be beaten or even alleviated through diet mean that most oncologists refuse to regard the high fat diet as a serious treatment option. However, Matthew Williams, a consultant clinical oncologist at Charing Cross Hospital in London, is something of an exception to this rule. 'There is evidence that, when combined with existing treatments, such as radiotherapy, it can improve them,' he says. 'And it may reduce side-effects.

But the only real data for that comes from rats. This is why I'm interested in running a human trial – to see if it translates. We have to be cautious about making claims because the rat brain is a poor model for human brains, and what works for rats often doesn't benefit humans. I certainly wouldn't recommend it was used on its own.'

But what about the individual success stories, such as Charles? 'The trouble is that they are the only ones we can talk to,' says Williams. 'There are others who followed the diet and died. Usually, we don't know if they did better or worse. The diet clearly doesn't work for everyone, but we don't yet know if it helps ten per cent or ninety per cent. That means we have to be very careful about who we put on it, because it is not a minor intervention. It involves a whole shift in your lifestyle, especially if you are in a family, and there are side-effects.'

At the time of writing, Williams was planning to address these issues by launching a small-scale trial on tolerability and quality of life. While this is certainly a welcome development, it is unlikely to convince his more sceptical colleagues, and we are probably still a long way from an irrefutable, large-scale study. 'In patients with aggressive brain tumours, a full trial to see if it improved survival would need about six hundred patients for the results to be considered reliable. That will be hard to do,' explains Williams.

Scepticism about the benefits of the diet among the oncology establishment isn't just related to the lack of trials. It also directly challenges conventional wisdom that cancer begins with random genetic mutations. However, this is only a hypothesis, so it may well be incorrect or at least only part of the story. Indeed, the US writer Travis Christofferson presented a convincing counter-argument in his 2015 book *Tripping over the Truth: How the Metabolic Theory of Cancer is Overturning One of Medicine's Most Entrenched Paradigms*. The book is based on Christofferson's research into the Cancer Genome Atlas – a database of the genes connected with cancer – and what he uncovered was startling. 'When the Atlas was launched,' he writes, 'the idea was that it would reveal an ordered sequence of maybe three to eight genes that when mutated would cause a particular type of cancer. Those genes would be an identifying signature of that cancer, like a fingerprint.' But what emerged was radically different. There were no predictable 'fingerprints'; instead, the mutations seemed to be almost entirely random. 'Those identified as starting and driving the cancer differed from person to person,' even those with precisely the same tumour type. Even more alarmingly, the mutations could be quite different in various cells of a single tumour. This meant that the dream of identifying particular mutations and then targeting each one with a specific drug was effectively over.

Senior researchers in America recognise this as a major problem. 'Something else is driving cancer; it's not just genes,' comments Bert Vogelstein, Director of the Ludwig Center and Clayton Professor of Oncology and Pathology at Johns Hopkins University. 'There is some dark matter in the genome that we can't detect.' Similarly, Nobel prizewinner and co-discoverer of DNA James Watson now believes that 'Further hundred-million-dollar annual injections [of cancer gene research funding] are not likely to produce the truly breakthrough drugs we so desperately need.'

Christofferson's book also explains why the theory that underpins the ketogenic diet – which relates to the way the body handles energy – fits the facts of cancer much better than the generally accepted hypothesis. Another Nobel prize winner, the German biochemist Otto Warburg, realised that cancer cells generate energy in a different way from healthy cells way back in the 1920s. Thereafter, further research established that the latter generate energy via their mitochondria. Essentially, healthy cells take glucose from the bloodstream and modify it into a substance known as pyruvate. This then travels through a channel in the mitochondria, where it is combined with oxygen – also drawn from the blood – to produce a chemical called ATP, which is the body's main unit of energy (see the illustration of how the body generates energy in Chapter 13, page 121).

By contrast, cancer cells have little or no ability to generate energy via their mitochondria. (It's not clear why this is the case, but it may have something to do with the fact that these cells undergo structural changes in the process of becoming cancerous.) Instead, they generate their ATP directly from glucose, which is almost eighty times less efficient than generating it from pyruvate. As a result, cancer cells need massive amounts of glucose. Indeed, this is why PET scans use radioactive glucose as a marker – it floods into the areas where cancerous tumours are growing.

As we know, the ketogenic diet drastically reduces the amount of glucose in the bloodstream, then the mitochondria of healthy cells use ketones to generate ATP. However, crucially, cancer cells cannot convert ketones into ATP. So, in effect, the diet specifically targets cancer cells while allowing healthy cells to keep functioning normally. This is in sharp contrast to conventional chemotherapy, which targets *all* of the body's fast-growing cells – healthy and cancerous alike – hence many of its unpleasant side effects. Moreover, as it drastically reduces a tumour's supply of fuel and therefore energy, the diet should make the cancer more vulnerable to chemotherapy. So, patients may need lower doses to achieve the same effect, and the side effects should be less severe. Dr Nelofer Syed, Senior Research Fellow and Lecturer in Cancer Biology at Imperial College London, is just one of an increasing number of advocates of this theory: 'Early research shows that the diet can improve the effectiveness of both chemotherapy and radiotherapy and that cancers find it difficult to use ketones for energy.' Her research also suggests that the ketogenic diet can make it difficult for tumours to hook up to a local blood supply, reduce inflammation and make it harder for the cancer to spread. In one paper, she and her colleagues conclude: 'Emerging data provides strong support for the use of the ketogenic diet in the treatment of malignant gliomas [brain cancers].'[27]

The diet also reduces the levels of the hormones insulin-like growth factor (IGF-1) and insulin as well as blood pressure – all of which are significant risk factors for cancer when they get too high. Moreover, it increases insulin sensitivity – meaning the hormone does its job better – by more than 70 per cent.[28] A further benefit relates to the diet's effect on so-called ROS (reactive oxygen species; also known as oxidants), which are normally kept in line by the body's own antioxidants, such as superoxide dismutase (SOD). Cancer cells can use ROS to help them grow, but they are killed by very high concentrations. Ketones push up ROS levels in tumours – as does chemotherapy – but, remarkably, actually reduce levels in healthy cells. They also sensitise tumours to chemotherapy, making them more responsive, while simultaneously reducing the toxic effects.

Ongoing research into the use of the ketogenic diet is essential because, frankly, traditional oncology's record is far from stellar. Indeed, in 2016, Peter Wise, a former consultant physician and senior lecturer, admitted: 'Chemotherapy drugs have had little effect on survival in adults with metastatic cancer.' For instance, a 2004 meta-study found that, 'For 90% of patients – including those with the commonest tumours of the lung, prostate, colon and breast – drug therapy increased five years survival by less than 2.5% – an overall survival benefit of around three months.' Moreover, 'The 48 new drug "regimens" approved by the American FDA between 2002 and 2014 had a median overall survival benefit of 2.1 months.'[29] Yet, the vast majority of cancer patients are still obliged to rely entirely on drugs, however modest the benefits and however harsh the side effects. Meanwhile, there is a stubborn reluctance to explore the potential of non-drug therapies, such as ketones. Is there any way to reconcile this conflict?

Well, in 2017, Professor Siddhartha Mukherjee – one of the biggest names in cancer research – made a suggestion.[30] His big idea was to focus on the body's metabolic system and ensure that it stayed cancer unfriendly. Rather than thinking of the disease as the creation of rogue mutations that should be targeted and eliminated, we need to think of cancer cells as members of an invasive species. They are not genetic packages containing all they need to multiply, but invaders whose success or failure is heavily influenced by the body's own defences. And those defences are directly linked to diet.

Japanese knotweed, a modest, easily controlled species in its native islands, transforms into a rampaging, voracious pest in British gardens simply because Britain lacks some of the inhibiting factors that keep it in line in Japan. The problem has nothing to do with the plant's genes. And the same is true for cancer. 'Ask not what cancer is doing to you,' Mukherjee wrote, 'but what you are doing to cancer.' The implication is that cancer needs to be treated from an ecological perspective: identify the conditions that allow it to flourish, then eliminate them.

Of course, this will require oncologists to adopt a radically different perspective. They will have to become familiar with 'invasion ecology' in order to investigate the many possible factors that may have allowed a species that was a well-behaved Dr Jekyll to become a Mr Hyde. Ecologists' tools include webs of nutrition, predation, climate and topography – all of which are subject to complex feedback loops.

Mukherjee didn't propose following a holistic approach to strengthen the body's defences. Rather, he advocated more conventional research focusing on boosting the body's immune system. But he certainly opened a door to more serious consideration of the merits of the ketogenic diet in cancer treatment.

Is a Ketogenic Diet the Right Approach for All Cancers?

It may well be that a full-blown ketogenic diet, especially one that is exclusively based on meat and dairy, is unsafe for some cancer patients. In particular, some researchers have suggested that animal products may be detrimental to patients with colon, prostate and breast cancer (see Chapter 21 for advice on how to switch to a more fish-based high-fat diet). Concerns have also been raised that some cancer cells – including melanomas and prostate cancer – are able to use ketones for their energy needs. More research is certainly needed in this area.

On the other hand, Valter Longo, Professor of Gerontology and Biological Science at the University of Southern California, found strong evidence that the high fat diet can significantly reduce the side effects of chemotherapy.[31] And there is mounting evidence that it has an impact on neurogliomas (also called glioblastomas) – particularly aggressive brain cancers. This could be due to the fact that brain cells function particularly well on ketones, whereas cancer cells find it difficult, if not impossible, to derive energy from these compounds.

Chapter 4

About Turn on High Fat and Heart Disease

Heart disease has been central to the low fat debate since the very beginning. Indeed, it was the primary concern of Ancel Keys when he overthrew the loose consensus that fat was a natural part of the human diet and arbitrarily advocated the low fat diet instead (see Chapter 1). However, his evidence for this shift was dubious, at best. Moreover, contradictory findings mysteriously disappeared, sometimes for decades.

Take the Minnesota Coronary Experiment. This was a rigorous five-year study involving 9,000 hospital patients who were given polyunsaturated vegetable oils in place of saturated fat under controlled conditions. The trial concluded in 1973, at precisely the time when Keys was preparing his case, but the results were not published – for reasons unknown – until 2016. The conclusion was that the new regime lowered cholesterol, but this did nothing to reduce deaths from heart disease.[32]

Unfortunately, the unnecessary switch to low fat led to a dramatic increase in the use of trans fats. Now widely recognised as harmful – and especially detrimental to heart health – these substances were introduced specifically to replace the 'dangerous' saturated fats that the baking industry had used for decades. Perhaps inevitably, heart disease rocketed in the two or three decades when trans fats were in widespread use.

In 2017, a year after the Minnesota Coronary Experiment finally saw the light of day, the results of another huge (and extremely expensive) seven-year investigation involving 135,335 people was published. The aim of the study was to determine if eating saturated fat reduced life expectancy or increased the risk of experiencing cardiovascular problems.[33] The conclusion was that it did neither. In fact, the researchers established that high fat diets *reduced* the risk of dying young or having a stroke. Yet, public health bodies have continued to demonise saturated fat and still instruct people to avoid it.

This stubborn refusal to blame anything other than fat and cholesterol in the fight against heart disease has meant that far more convincing approaches have been ignored for half a century. Recently, though, some of the high fat pioneers have drawn attention to a much more plausible culprit: insulin.

It has long been acknowledged that diagnosed diabetics have a far greater risk of suffering heart disease than non-diabetics. However, there are also vast numbers of undiagnosed diabetics – some estimates suggest that they may comprise 60 per cent of the population – with high levels of insulin in their bloodstreams. As we shall see later, there is increasing evidence that the prevalence of this hormone throughout the population is driving the heart disease epidemic. Yet, cardiac patients are not routinely tested for raised insulin levels. In part, this is due to the medical establishment's unflinching adherence to the cholesterol theory. So, before we turn our attention to insulin, let's take a look at cholesterol and the use of statins to reduce it.

The Cholesterol Myth

Critics of the cholesterol theory, such as Dr Malcolm Kendrick,[34] have assembled a detailed and convincing case against it, yet it remains central to the treatment of heart disease around the world, seemingly regardless of mounting evidence against its efficacy. For instance, one Japanese study found that the mortality rate actually *declined* as the level of LDL – so-called 'bad cholesterol' – increased. Moreover, 'The same relationship exists among the elderly in all countries worldwide.'[35]

The standard means to reduce cholesterol – and therefore supposedly treat or prevent heart disease – is with statins. This has made them the most highly prescribed drugs around the world; currently, around seven million people take statins in the UK alone. Yet their proven benefits, especially with regard to prevention of heart disease, are negligible. In addition, there are increasing concerns about their side effects.

Nevertheless, statins' supporters, notably the Cholesterol Treatment Trialists (CTT) Collaboration organisation, based in Oxford, has continued to champion the drug. However, the independence of the CTT has come under increasing scrutiny. The organisation has been publishing largely favourable meta-analyses of the data from company-run trials since the early 1990s when it was given all the raw data from 28 large randomised statin trials, on the condition that they were not made available to independent researchers.

It is well established that company-run trials are considerably more likely to produce favourable results, and allowing non-company researchers access the raw data is now a fundamental principle of evidence-based medicine.[36]

Concern about the reliability of the CTT data on statin side effects, were raised by independent researchers in two BMJ articles which the director of CTT demanded be retracted. This triggered an investigation by an independent committee.[37]

One of its surprising findings was that, contrary to long-standing claims that the CTT was funded by charities and independent bodies, it had received over £268 million in funding from Merck – manufacturer of the world's best-selling statin.[38] The head of the CTT later admitted that he and his team had never even looked for information about side effects in the trials data.[39]

Insulin – the True Culprit

Challenging entrenched medical opinion – not to mention the financial clout of the global pharmaceutical industry – is a pretty daunting prospect, but a handful of brave souls have put their heads above the parapet. One such is Dr Thomas Dayspring, Chief Academic Officer at True Health Diagnostics. He has given many talks and interviews on social media in which he makes it clear that he regards LDL as a near-worthless predictor for cardiovascular issues. A far better indicator, he claims, is insulin resistance linked to a high carbohydrate diet. For these patients, he argues, other markers of raised risk include a raised level of fats in the blood (triglycerides), rising blood pressure and inflammation. He can be seen analysing heart risk data in a fascinating video interview (see Resources page 360).

Another US physician – Jeffry Gerber – has been running insulin tests on his cardiovascular patients for years.[40] 'We've done two thousand tests on glucose and insulin on patients at risk for heart problems over the last seventeen years,' he says. 'Many of them have what I call "metabolic mayhem", so just focusing on lowering calories and cholesterol and fat misses the mark.' Gerber insists that there is a 'strong relationship between hyperinsulinemia and heart disease ... but you won't find it if you don't test for it. Furthermore, running a regular glucose tolerance test isn't enough, because you can have normal glucose but a sky-high level of insulin to keep it that way.' It's a similar situation to when a car seems to be running normally, but in reality it is using gallons of oil to stop the engine seizing up. Checking the body's insulin level is exactly the same as checking the oil level in your car – if it's not where it should be, you've got a serious problem.

The clinician who first established this link between insulin and heart disease was Joseph Kraft, a pathologist at St Joseph's Hospital, Chicago. In the early 1970s, he started to explore the connection between the levels of glucose and insulin in the bloodstream. At the time, it was generally assumed that they rose and fell in parallel to each other: as glucose increased after eating carbohydrates, the pancreas released extra insulin to clear away any excess that wasn't needed for energy; then, as the glucose dropped, so did the insulin. However, nobody had actually bothered to measure the level of insulin. Kraft did just that – in 3,650 patients – and the results were startling. Half of those who had 'normal' levels of glucose had insulin levels that would qualify them as diabetic.[41] The obvious implication was that diabetes was being massively under-diagnosed ... especially when Kraft later revised his figure from 50 per cent to 70 per cent![42] And, as we have seen, diabetes is one of the main risk factors for heart disease.

Later research established precisely why excessive insulin is likely to cause heart disease. Basically, it does serious damage to the arteries. These blood vessels have a lining called the endothelium, which plays a major role in controlling blood clotting, flow and pressure. In turn, the endothelium is coated with a slippery, gel-like substance called glycocalyx, which is equally important for heart health, as it controls the flow of hormones and red blood cells. However, a very high level of insulin prevents the glycocalyx from releasing nitric oxide, meaning that the arteries are left with no protection against high blood pressure. It also seems to make the blood more likely to coagulate – a key factor in heart disease. Finally, one study found that antioxidants mitigate the arterial damage, which suggests that high insulin levels also promote the release of harmful oxidants.[43] Therefore, while testing for insulin – as well as glucose – now seems a prerequisite for accurate diagnosis of diabetes, it might be equally valuable in identifying patients who are at risk of developing heart disease.[44]

Years of a high carbohydrate diet, which creates regular spikes in blood glucose each and every day, is one of the main drivers of high insulin levels and insulin resistance. The muscles, liver and fat cells, where excess glucose is usually stored, demand the release of ever more insulin before they respond and accept delivery. This is common knowledge in the diabetes world, but almost never considered as a risk factor for heart disease, even though a group of researchers concluded that insulin resistance is a 'powerful' predictor of cardiovascular problems as long ago as 2002.[45] The previous year, another study had established that patients with low insulin levels are less likely to develop a range of age-related disorders, including heart disease, stroke, cancer and diabetes.[46]

These findings suggested that the holy grail of cardiology – an accurate test to identify patients at high risk of developing heart disease – was within our grasp. The equation is simple: high insulin equals increased susceptibility to heart disease. 'We live in an insulin-boosting world,' says Ivor Cummings, an Irish engineer who designed his own programme to tackle heart disease and now talks persuasively about the urgent need for widespread insulin testing.[47] 'Many things can raise your insulin levels besides a poor diet, lack of exercise, obesity and getting older. These include stress, smoking and lack of sleep. In fact, the seventy per cent figure is probably an underestimate of the number of people with high insulin who are heading for a heart attack. Tragedies could be stopped twenty years early with a simple blood test – the fasting insulin test.' Your GP is unlikely to order one of these potentially life-saving tests on the NHS, but online kits are available (see Resources, page 368).

The medical fraternity's reluctance to introduce testing for high insulin may be due to the fact that most cardiologists do not consider diet as a 'proper' treatment for heart disease. But there is increasing evidence that a low carb, high fat diet (and/or a low GL diet; see Part 2) is actually the *best* way to prevent and treat heart disease.

Another possibility, rarely mentioned in cardiology circles, is that high insulin and glucose levels transform cholesterol in a process known as glycosylation. Diabetics are probably already familiar with this term, as their red blood cells are constantly glycosylated. And the greater the glycosylation, the more they experience glucose spikes. Similarly, while we are repeatedly told that normal cholesterol is the major villain in heart disease, a recent study failed to establish any link between it and coronary atherosclerosis. By contrast, the researchers concluded that high levels of glucose and *glycosylated* cholesterol, effectively sugar damaged cholesterol, were 'of high importance' in the development of heart disease.[48] This may be because macrophages – white blood cells that are the main strike force of the body's immune system – engulf the glycosylated cholesterol and turn into fat-laden 'foam' cells. These cells are found in arterial plaque, which causes the blockages that lead to heart attacks.

Low Carb, High Fat – a Good Strategy against Heart Disease

It seems that high glucose and insulin levels are major – but seriously neglected – risk factors in the development of heart problems. But is the ketogenic diet really the best way to address these issues? After all, for decades, the public health authorities have insisted that heart attacks are directly linked to the consumption of saturated fat.

Yet, in 2014, a study involving more than 80,000 women found that there was no increased risk of heart disease after three years on a low carb diet. Moreover, such a diet may 'moderately reduce the risk of coronary heart disease' when vegetable rather than animal sources of fat and protein are eaten.[49] (See Chapter 24 for more information on the benefits of vegetable protein.) In addition, a series of trials between 1996 and 2013 found that the high fat diet not only aided weight loss but also counteracted cardiovascular risk factors.[50]

One of the most common concerns about the high fat, low carb diet is the effect it might have over the long term, especially when one of the more challenging ketogenic versions is followed. However, at least one study offers considerable reassurance. A group of ten epilepsy patients were placed on a ketogenic diet and their progress was monitored over the course of ten years. The diet helped to alleviate their symptoms and 'No cardiovascular risks were identified.'[51]

Chapter 5

Eat Fat to Lose Weight

If you want to lose weight, then the low carb, high fat diet is just about the best way to do it. And it's safe, despite all the scare stories. So you can say goodbye to sweets, cakes and puddings, bread, pasta and rice, and starchy vegetables, like potatoes and parsnips. Instead, you will be eating a diet of mostly unprocessed, very healthy food. Your meals will be delicious and varied, and they will contain copious amounts of fat and protein from meat (mostly white rather than red), fish, eggs, raw nuts and seeds, cream, butter, cheese and full-fat milk, plenty of green leafy vegetables, such as cauliflower, cabbage, broccoli and Brussels sprouts, as well as natural plant oils from coconuts, avocados and olives.

In this chapter, we will explain why this diet is so effective for weight loss, outline how to keep track of how your body is responding to it, and suggest some supplements that might increase the efficiency of the ketogenic machine you have activated.

The first step is to change the proportions of the three macronutrients. Fat must provide 65–80 per cent of your daily calories (see Chapter 22 for more details), with protein providing 20–25 per cent and carbohydrates just 5–10 per cent. We allow for a certain amount of wiggle room because everyone responds differently to the three macronutrients.

At first sight, you may find these percentages alarming. On the other hand, they may seem strangely familiar, especially if you have previously tried the Atkins diet. Back in the 1990s, the media presented that diet as a golden ticket to eat as much steak, sausages and bacon as you liked, as long as you consumed only 20–30g of carbs each day. (In reality, Atkins recommended this approach for only the first few months. Thereafter, carb intake could gradually increase to 100g a day.) Also, while the diet certainly seemed to be an effective way to lose weight, there were countless reports of dog breath and dire warnings from dietitians about excess protein and kidney damage. Nevertheless, at the time, millions tried it and sang its praises (although a large proportion of them subsequently regained the weight).

Few of the advocates of Atkins knew that it was largely a rehash of a diet that dated all the way back to 1863. In that year, a corpulent London undertaker named William Banting published a pamphlet in which he explained that he had lost several stones simply by cutting out sugary, starchy carbs. It was a bestseller and the diet became a mainstay of medical textbooks until the 1970s, when it was ousted by a new, radical alternative – the low fat diet.

So, the high fat approach is nothing new, and the medical establishment had no issues with it for more than a century. Moreover, as we have seen, it has proved highly effective as a treatment for severe epilepsy over the course of many decades. Even so, the argument continues to rage over whether it is more effective than the low fat diet when the aim is simply to lose weight.

Evidence for the Benefits of the High Fat Approach

A recent review of the evidence by Professor Timothy Noakes, mentioned earlier, a sports scientist and campaigner for low carb diets at the University of Cape Town, found that high fat diets repeatedly performed as well or better than the low fat alternatives in terms of weight loss.[52] For instance, in a year-long study of 148 obese men and women, one group's diet was set at 55 per cent carbohydrates (150g), while those in the second group were restricted to less than 40g of carbs each day, but allowed to eat as much fat and protein as they liked. By the end of the trial, the second group had lost an average of 5.3kg and reduced their body fat by 1.3 per cent, while those in the first group had lost just 1.8kg, and their body fat had *increased* by 0.3 per cent.[53]

A second trial involving 34 overweight or obese diabetics reported very similar results. One group was put on a standard low fat, calorie-restricted diet, which provided 150g of carbohydrates per day. The others went on a high fat diet with no more than 50g of carbs per day – a sufficiently small intake to put them into ketosis. Both groups were taught about diet and learned psychological techniques to help them change their behaviour. After three months those in the low fat group had lost an average of 2.6kg, whereas those in the high fat group had lost 5.5kg. In addition, 44 per cent of the second group had been able to reduce their medication, compared with only 11 per cent in the first group.[54]

In both of these trials, the low fat groups cut their calorific intake by at least 500 calories a day, whereas the second (high fat) groups did not. Yet, the 'eat as much as you like' groups lost twice as much weight as the calorie-restricted groups.

This finding directly contradicts the official explanation for obesity: that it is due to eating too much. On the other hand, it correlates precisely with the 'Carbohydrate–Insulin Model of Obesity', developed by Professor David Ludwig of Boston's

Children's Hospital (see Chapter 13 for more details).[55] Ludwig points out that something rather surprising happens if you try to overfeed people in order to make them put on weight: our bodies react by increasing the amount of energy they use and dampening down the hunger response, so there is more likelihood of *losing* weight.[56]

Glucose, Fat and Ketones – Three Very Different Sources of Energy

As we saw earlier, when a body is deprived of carbohydrates, the blood glucose that is normally used to power the brain and the muscles starts to drop almost immediately, along with the level of insulin. The body's natural response is to release fat into the bloodstream to meet its immediate energy requirements. This is why we start to lose weight after only a couple of days on a low *carb* diet. By contrast, insulin and glucose levels remain pretty much the same on a low *fat* diet, so little or no fat is released from storage and little or no weight is lost. Moreover, a 2012 study found that people on a low carb diet burned around 300 extra calories each day ... while resting! According to the researchers, 'that equals the number of calories typically burned in an hour of moderate-intensity physical activity'.[57]

This situation is fine for the muscles, as they are able to process the released fat to meet all of their energy needs. However, the brain is unable to extract energy from fat. This might seem to be a serious design flaw, especially as our bodies can store no more than 300g of glucose (in the form of glycogen), and the brain uses about 100g each day. So, why does it not shut down after three days, after those reserves of glucose have run out? The answer is ketones, which the liver manufactures from the released fat that is now circulating around the bloodstream as well as ingested fats, such as MCT oil (see Chapter 19). The brain can process these little packets of energy – in fact, it may prefer them to glucose – and they provide all the fuel it needs to keep functioning perfectly. As an added bonus, the body simply pees out any ketones that it doesn't use; they are not converted back into fat, in marked contrast to unused glucose.

A Few Words of Advice about Ketogenic Diets

People on high fat diets work with their bodies rather than against them. But that's not to say that the first few days are easy. First, after years of large daily doses of carbohydrate, your body is effectively addicted to them. (Don't worry: we'll show you how to break this addiction in Chapter 16.) Second, you have been exposed to decades of propaganda about the dangers of saturated fat – such as that it will make you obese and clog your arteries – yet you are about to consume large quantities of it. That's a significant psychological hurdle to overcome. Third, it might be three weeks before your body is fully 'keto adapted' – that is, able to meet all of its energy needs through fat and ketones rather than glucose. Fourth, during the first phase of the change-over (which normally lasts no more than three to four days), you may experience so-called 'keto flu' – various mildly unpleasant side-effects, including low energy, headaches and melancholia. Just try to remember that your body is making a lot of adjustments and you'll get through it.

One thing you won't have to worry about is hunger, because you can eat as much fat as you want, whenever you want. There's no need to stick to set meal times; listen to your body instead. You will soon find yourself eating much less than before, precisely because you are not as hungry as you were on the standard low fat, calorie-controlled diet. And that's great for weight loss.

You are likely to lose 3–5lb (1–2kg) very quickly, but most of that will be due to water loss as your body extracts glucose from your stores of glycogen.[58] You'll put it back on almost immediately if you stop the diet, so you'll need to persevere if you want more permanent results by breaking down the body's reserves of fat. Once you've reached your target weight, you may want to exit ketosis and start to increase your intake of carbs, but you should ensure that these are slow carbs (see Part 2), as changing your diet in this way will keep your glucose and insulin at healthy levels, which in turn will make a rebound weight gain much less likely.

Monitoring Your Diet

When you embark on the high fat diet, it might be an idea to invest in a monitor to keep track of your progress. Currently, only diabetics routinely check their insulin and glucose levels, but these measurements are also accurate indicators of whether the body is in or out of ketosis. Otherwise, it can be difficult to tell one way or the other. There are a number of relatively cheap monitors on the market, some of which measure glucose and/or insulin from a pinprick of blood, while others use a 'stick' that detects ketones in urine. Another device measures the ketone levels in your breath. Sometimes, the results can be surprising. For instance, it's not unusual for people to assume that they have been in ketosis for months only to discover that they haven't been close. (See Chapter 26 for more information on monitoring.)

When you enter ketosis, your ketone level will register 0.5mmol/l before increasing to 1–4mmol/l. At that point, you will be in the most effective state for weight loss as long as your glucose level (also measured in mmol/l) is also less than 5. It's easy to drop out of ketosis if you are not careful about your carb intake, but regular monitoring will allow you to rectify this immediately if it starts to happen, either by eliminating the carbs or by fasting (see Chapter 15). A monitor is also useful if you want to experiment with supplementing exogenous (from outside the body) ketones.

A Little Help from Outside

Supplements usually come in the form of a powder or an oil that can be added to shakes or smoothies. Then there are the three types of natural ketones. First off, the liver's production line is acetoacetate (AcAc), some of which gets turned into the main ketone workhorse beta-hydroxybutyrate (BHB). One the big pluses of ketones for weight loss is that if you make too many, they don't get stored as fat; instead they break down into a simpler form, acetone, and are breathed out.

All of the supplements, such as C8 oil, contain BHB rather than AcAc, and they are all designed to accelerate the process of entering or re-entering ketosis (see Chapter 19 for more information). They also reduce hunger pangs, so they can be useful during intermittent or alternate-day fasts.

In addition to supplementing your diet with exogenous ketones, you may well benefit from taking a few extra vitamins and minerals, as these have key roles to play in many crucial ketosis processes (see Chapter 25 for further details). For instance, vitamin C helps the cells' mitochondria to turn glucose, fat and ketones into energy. Similarly, the B vitamins niacin and its cousin NAD (nicotinamide adenine dinucleotide) help to transport ketones into the mitochondria. However, the body's natural reserves of NAD decline as we age, and ketosis increases the body's demand, so it is a good idea to supplement it during a high fat diet. The same is true of another B vitamin – biotin – which is critical for the metabolism of ketones. Finally, the amino acid carnitine is a vital component in two processes: burning fat and turning it into ketones. Therefore, supplementing will help you to maximise your conversion of fat into energy and eliminate the possibility of falling into carnitine deficiency – a serious condition that can result in muscle weakness, fatigue and irritability, among a host of other symptoms.

Chapter 6

Your Brain Needs Fat

As we have seen, muscle cells are well equipped to burn fat for energy, whereas brain cells – neurons – are not. There are so many neurons – some 100 billion of them – packed into such a small area that there isn't any free space, so they have to use the cleanest, fastest, most efficient fuel, rather than inefficient fat. Usually this is glucose, but when the glucose 'engine' starts to malfunction, as often happens with diabetics, ketones are a terrific alternative source of energy for the brain. And there is growing evidence that they have benefits for non-diabetics, too.

In 2011, a Florida-based paediatrician named Mary Newport published a book with the provocative title *Alzheimer's Disease: What if There Was a Cure?* She was writing from deep personal experience, as her husband had been battling dementia for some time. Mainstream Alzheimer's researchers and charities ignored the book, but this was hardly surprising as the central idea seemed eccentric and fanciful. Newport's claim was that several daily doses of coconut oil had arrested her husband's inexorable decline into severe early-onset Alzheimer's.

At the time, the assumption – in the Western world, at least – was that coconut oil must be dangerous because it contains high levels of saturated fat. Moreover, sceptics pointed out that billions of pounds had already been spent on pharmaceutical research, so it was hardly likely that the answer to Alzheimer's lay with the humble coconut. These counter-arguments all seemed very rational and based on rigorous science, yet there is still no sign of the pharmaceutical industry coming up with an effective treatment. In the meantime, though, many Americans have made coconut oil a basic component of their diet because, as Newport pointed out, it helps the body to generate ketones. And ketones provide the fuel that dementia patients' brains so desperately need.

Professor Kieran Clarke (whom we met in the Introduction) and Dr Richard Veech, a biochemist at the American National Institutes of Health, were two of just a handful of senior scientists who felt that Newport's claims merited further investigation. 'When a supply of ketones arrives in a brain that is having problems with making use of the glucose that normally fuels neurons, it automatically switches over to being able to use them,' says Clarke. 'It behaves rather like a hybrid car, working with whatever fuel is available.' Another supporter is Professor Stephen Cunnane of Sherbrooke University in Canada, an expert on fatty acid metabolism in the brain who has held the 'Canada Research Chair on Dietary Fatty Acids and Cognitive Function during Ageing'. In a recent paper he and his colleagues explored whether ketones can 'help rescue brain fuel supply in later life'.[59]

Mary Newport's book delivered a message of hope. Her husband had been deteriorating for years by the time he started taking daily doses of coconut oil. Thereafter, though, 'The transformation was remarkable. He started exercising again, he was able to read – things he hadn't done for four years. His conversation improved; he even got his libido back. An MRI scan showed his brain had stopped shrinking.'

Is Alzheimer's Brain Diabetes?

If Newport's claims are true, and dementia patients' brains do indeed benefit from switching from glucose to ketones as their main fuel supply, we need to establish why this is the case. One recent theory suggests that Alzheimer's should be considered as a form of diabetes of the brain, so, like diabetes itself, treatment should focus on reducing the body's levels of insulin and glucose. This makes sense, as diabetics are three times more likely to develop Alzheimer's than non-diabetics.

Stephen Cunnane explains, 'The brain has the greatest demand for fuel of any organ in the body and evolutionarily ketones emerged to ensure that the brain's rapacious demand had a greater chance of being met. This source of fuel may also have been a factor allowing for the threefold expansion of the brain around two million years ago that is associated with all our highly developed cognitive abilities.' Cunnane adds that ketones are still vital for wiring up the human brain during infancy: 'They are produced from MCTs [medium-chain triglycerides] in mothers' milk, and even when babies stop breastfeeding, they remain in ketosis at much higher levels than adults for the first year of their lives.'[60] Indeed, it is estimated that ketones meet half of the energy needs of an infant's brain, precisely at the time when the organ is expanding at a furious rate and demanding massive amounts of fuel.

Babies can survive on the ketones that their livers produce from their own fat reserves for as long as sixty days; and, interestingly, even a high carb diet doesn't push them out of ketosis. Given this preference for ketones during construction of the brain at the beginning of life, it makes sense that the same fuel is equally beneficial towards the end, especially in those areas of the brain that are involved in memory and cognition.

Professor Cunnane's research has shown that Alzheimer's patients start to suffer glucose deficiency in certain regions of the brain even before they start to experience any symptoms. There may be various reasons for this, including low grade infections, which increase the immune system's demands for glucose, and insulin resistance, which makes it more difficult for the fuel to make its way into the neurons. 'We know from our scanning research that the glucose deficit is not due to damage to the neurons, but to insufficient amounts being available as fuel,' explains Cunnane. 'It's safe to treat this deficiency with ketones.' On the other hand, if the condition remains untreated, the fuel-deprived neurons suffer the sort of damage that ultimately leads to Alzheimer's.

Even though the full-blown ketogenic diet is a highly effective means to generate the ketones that the brain can use in place of glucose, it may not be advisable for sufferers of dementia. 'If I had brain cancer or diabetes, or I wanted to lose weight, I'd go on the diet without hesitation,' says Cunnane. 'But it involves big changes to something very familiar, which can distress Alzheimer's patients.' It was for this reason that Mary Newport experimented with coconut oil, rather than placing her husband on a radically different, high fat diet. Because the oil contains MCTs, the liver can convert it directly into ketones without any need to follow a strict low carb diet.[61]

The Miracle of Coconut Oil

Newport's husband had been declining steadily for four years by the time she decided to give coconut oil a try. His mini-mental state examination (MMSE) had dropped from 23 to 12 (30 is normal), and an MMR brain scan found a pattern of brain shrinkage that is typical among Alzheimer's patients. In light of these results, no one expected anything other than further decline.

Newport started with a modest dose of 35ml (two tablespoons) of coconut oil once a day before gradually increasing the amount. She then added three tablespoons of purified MCT oil (see Chapter 19) for every four tablespoons of coconut oil until her husband was getting a total of 165ml a day, delivered in three or four servings. This combination provided a steady supply of fuel because, while the liver finds it easy to convert the C8-rich MCT oil into ketones, most are gone from the body in just three hours, whereas coconut oil provides fewer ketones, but they last for up to eight hours. After three months on this regime, her husband's MMSE test results had increased to 20 and his mood had improved significantly.

As Stephen Cunnane explains, while coconut oil delivers a relatively modest amount of ketones (certainly in comparison with MCT oil), it seems to have a disproportionately large positive effect. It's not quite clear why this is the case, but 'it could be because of its antibacterial properties, which can help to combat the various infections that affect elderly people and can divert energy from the brain to the immune system'.

Unfortunately, the optimism of the first few months dissipated as Newport's husband started to decline again. However, she was not yet ready to throw in the towel, so she obtained some of the synthetic ketones that Kieran Clarke had recently developed. 'It was like turning on a switch,' Newport says. 'We gave him a dose in the morning when he seemed in a fog and he was soon much more alert and very much aware of what was going on around him. Then his condition deteriorated through the day, as if his brain was going dark again. In the evening, we'd give him another dose and he'd come back, but when he woke the next morning he needed another dose because he was confused again. It was a very clear demonstration that although his brain was unable to use glucose for fuel, it could still use ketones.'

Incredibly, these intriguing results failed to spark any mainstream interest in the use of synthetic ketones, and at the time of writing they were still virtually unknown in the UK. They are licensed in the United States, but very expensive and mostly used by elite athletes to improve performance. A price drop, coupled with some large-scale scientific trials, might transform the way that Alzheimer's is treated around the world. Yet, research into the benefits of ketones is still in its infancy and hampered by a lack of funding. This is scandalous, because the few trials that have been conducted suggest that ketones' benefits aren't limited to providing extra fuel for neurons that are starved of glucose. They also seem to protect the brain from further damage and might even play a role in repairing it.

Animal studies suggest that ketones reduce the bundles of tangled nerves – known as tau – that are found in the brains of people with Alzheimer's while also lowering inflammation and repairing damaged mitochondria. Moreover, they seem to offer some protection against harmful oxidants, which the mitochondria release as waste products during the process of energy production.

Of course, ketones should not be seen as a panacea for dementia, and more research is needed, but we know that they have been a valuable source of fuel for the human brain for millions of years, so it would be remarkable if they weren't beneficial in a number of significant ways. Unfortunately, though, the medical establishment has shown a lamentable reluctance to explore those potential benefits. For instance, in 2018, Alzheimer's Research UK responded to the question 'Can coconut oil help?' as follows: 'We can't be sure. There is preliminary research into some components of coconut oil, but so far, the research is inconclusive. The most important thing when considering a complementary therapy is to talk to your doctor because these products can interact with normal medication.' Yet that 'normal medication' does not have a great track record itself. The most widely used brand in the treatment of dementia – Aricept – has some serious potential side effects including nausea, diarrhoea and slow heart rhythms that can lead to fainting. Moreover, even the manufacturer admits that it is often effective for no more than six months.

The Value of Vitamins and Minerals

Alzheimer's patients' metabolism starts to fail long before their symptoms become apparent. Many have high levels of the toxic amino acid homocysteine, which can cause damage to the brain. However, this can be combated by taking high doses of B vitamins and omega-3 fats, with the result that memory decline is either arrested or halted altogether.[62] (Several studies have claimed to disprove the benefits of B vitamins, but all of these gave either low doses or high doses to people with normal levels of homocysteine who had no room for improvement.[63]) Stephen Cunnane suggests that supplementing omega-3, iron, iodine, zinc, copper and B vitamins might help to reverse some of the symptoms of dementia and increase the resilience of patients' metabolic systems.

The researcher who has gone furthest in assembling a package of lifestyle changes to stave off Alzheimer's is Professor Dale Bredesen, a neurologist at the University of California, Los Angeles. His programme advocates getting sufficient sleep, reducing stress, following various diets and adhering to a strict exercise regime. Early results among a thousand volunteers have been highly promising.

A High Fat Ketogenic Diet Can Counteract Epilepsy

As we saw earlier, the ketogenic diet has long been a standard treatment for childhood epilepsy. Indeed, the benefits of this approach have been well known for about a hundred years.[64] However, it was 2008 before Professor Helen Cross, a neurologist and expert in childhood epilepsy at Great Ormond Street Hospital, London, ran the first rigorous scientific trial. Unsurprisingly, this proved what many neurologists had known all along: that a high fat diet is a highly effective treatment for epilepsy.

'About thirty per cent of epileptic children don't respond to the drugs and they can have a dreadful time: a hundred fits a day is not uncommon,' says Susan Wood, a registered dietitian who works for Matthew's Friends Clinics, a registered charity that advocates the introduction of the ketogenic diet for all sufferers of the condition. It's still not exactly clear why this diet is so effective, but it probably has something to do with the fact that it turns off the master switch (mTOR) that controls how much energy our bodies can use (see Chapter 13 for more details) and reduces the activity of one of the excitatory chemicals in the brain (glutamate). Simply reducing carbs also seems to have an anti-seizure effect, while changes in the neurons' mitochondria may be involved, too. Moreover, a recent study in the *Lancet* found that MCT oil (which is often taken as part of the diet) has some significant direct effects, such as blocking glutamate receptors and increasing the amount of energy that is available to neurons by boosting their mitochondria.[65]

Unfortunately, the ketogenic diet is sometimes accompanied by a range of unpleasant side effects, especially in the first few days, such as vomiting, constipation, heartburn, tiredness and even a temporary increase in the number of seizures. However, these are often mitigated by extensive supplementation, including: a general multivitamin with minerals plus omega-3 for general health; laxatives for constipation; additional selenium, magnesium, zinc, phosphorous and vitamin D for possible heart issues; and carnitine, which can help with seizures and low energy levels.[66]

Given that children with epilepsy are known to benefit from following a ketogenic diet, it seems reasonable to assume that adult epileptics would find the approach similarly beneficial. However, as is so often the case, this has not been properly tested, as yet.

The Potential Benefits of High Fat Diets among Patients with Parkinson's Disease

In light of the profound effect that the ketogenic diet has on the structure and workings of the brain, it is plausible to suggest that it might prove useful in the treatment of Parkinson's disease. All of the studies in this area are still in their early stages, but some of the initial results are promising.

Parkinson's patients have insufficient amounts of the neuro-transmitter dopamine, and at present they are routinely treated with an amino acid named L-dopa. However, for it to work, the neurons' mitochondria need to be able to generate sufficient energy to turn it into dopamine. As we know, the mitochondria are usually powered by glucose that is extracted from carbohydrates, but if this process isn't working well – and there is evidence that this is often the case among Parkinson's patients – the ketones produced during ketosis could be extremely beneficial.

One recent trial placed one group of patients on a low fat, high carb diet and another group on a ketogenic diet for a period of eight weeks.[67] Those on the latter diet showed a 41 per cent improvement in behaviour and mood, compared with only an 11 per cent improvement among those on the low fat diet. The high carb group also experienced more hunger, while some of those on the ketogenic diet suffered a slight and occasional worsening of tremors and/or muscle rigidity.

Parkinson's experts Geoffrey and Lucille Leader point out that certain amino acids compete for absorption with the standard medication for the condition, so some protein-rich foods should not be eaten within two hours of taking the medication. (The

Leaders explain their approach in detail in their book *Parkinson's Disease: Reducing Symptoms with Nutrition and Drugs*.[68]) Therefore, supplementing exogenous ketones either alongside or shortly after medication, while avoiding protein-rich foods, certainly seems to merit a trial.

Part 2

Slow Carbs Rule

We all have two engines that run on two completely different types of fuel: ketones and glucose. In Part 1, we explored the benefits of running on ketones. In this part, we explore the benefits of running on glucose ... but the *right kind* of glucose: that is, slow carbs, not fast carbs.

Chapter 7

Not All Carbs Are Created Equal

Having read Part 1, you might be feeling pretty down about carbs. However, it is important to remember that not all 'sugars' in carbs behave in the same way. So, while a low carb, ketogenic diet can certainly aid weight loss and help in the fight against diabetes, heart disease or even cancer, a low glycemic load diet, based on eating the right kind of carbohydrates in the right quantities, may be just as effective.

I (Patrick) have been championing a low glycemic load diet since 1987, and have seen significant weight loss – as well as dramatic improvements in patients with diabetes and heart disease – as a result. So, it is music to my ears that increasing numbers of doctors are finally joining the low carb revolution.

My first venture into this world focused on promoting foods with a low 'glycemic index' (GI) – a term coined by Thomas Wolever and David Jenkins (now Professor of Nutrition at the University of Toronto) in the 1980s. GI is a 'quality only' measure in that it tells you precisely how fast a certain food raises your blood sugar. However, the real magic started to happen when I combined the right *quantity* of carbs with the right *quality* to calculate a food's glycemic load (GL). Unfortunately, despite more than three decades of consistently positive research findings on the benefits of a low GL diet, conventional medical advice – such as the recommendations of the National Institute for Health and Care Excellence (NICE) – does not even acknowledge GL's existence. As a result, rates of obesity, diabetes, hormonal cancers, heart disease and dementia continue to rise.

Later, we will explore the ways in which a low GL diet prevents and/or reverses all of these illnesses. First, though, we need to explain precisely how carbs work and why they should not always be viewed as the devil incarnate.

The Bitter Truth about Sugar

Under normal circumstances, glucose – rather than fat – is clearly the human body's favourite fuel. While it takes an average of four days to start burning ketones for energy, it takes only four minutes to switch back to burning glucose. Our complex metabolism is perfectly designed to transform carbohydrates into glucose, and then to liberate the boundless energy that is contained within this supercharged molecule – an amazing process takes place in each and every cell's mitochondria.

So, what's the problem, given that our bodies have evolved to be highly efficient glucose-burning machines? For the answer, we need to go on a journey into the world of carbs and learn why not all sugars are equal. Once you understand the dynamics, it will soon become obvious what you should eat in order to stay healthy.

Our livers cleverly convert the predominant sugar in fruit – fructose – into glucose, a process that is similar to turning diesel into petrol. The sort of sugar that many people still put in their tea – pure, white and deadly – is sucrose, which is made up of one unit of glucose and one unit of fructose. In the body, an enzyme splits these compounds apart to liberate the glucose and give you an instant hit of both sweetness and energy, but you need another three enzyme steps, all of which occur in the liver, to turn the fructose into more glucose. This is why blood glucose levels increase at a slower rate after eating fructose than they do after eating either glucose itself or sucrose. It just takes longer.

Other common sugars include lactose (milk sugar), maltose (grain sugar) and xylose (the predominant sugar in berries, cherries and plums). The latter is actually a sugar-alcohol which, while tasting sweet, has very little effect on either blood glucose level or the release of insulin. Indeed, one teaspoon of sucrose has the same effect on your blood glucose level as nine teaspoons of xylose (xylitol in its crystallised form).

So, not all sugars are equal, which means that your blood glucose level and insulin release depend on *two* key aspects of the food you eat:

- How many carbs are available – quantity.
- And how quickly those carbs will raise your glucose level – quality.

Focusing on only one of these can be very misleading.

A food's 'quality' is expressed in terms of its GI, which is linked to the amount of time it takes the body to convert the sugar into glucose. Therefore, glucose itself has a GI of 100 per cent. By contrast, fructose is just 16 per cent, while sucrose (white table sugar) is 65 per cent. Many low carb, high fat diets, which aim to push the body into ketosis, focus solely on the quantity of carbs, for instance by advocating no more than 30g, 50g or 100g of available carbohydrate each day, regardless of type. ('Available' is shorthand for 'available to turn into glucose', because indigestible fibre, a kind of carbohydrate that the body cannot convert into glucose, doesn't count.) Meanwhile, many low GI diets neglect the quantity side of the equation and concentrate exclusively on quality, for instance by suggesting you can eat as much fructose-rich food as you like. Either way, they tell only half the story.

Problems with the Low GI Approach

Unfortunately, if you were to eat nothing but a whole load of low GI foods, you might still end up with blood sugar problems. Moreover, you might unnecessarily eliminate a range of healthy foods, such as fruit, simply because they are rated high GI.

Take the following meal: carrot (92 GI) and pumpkin (75 GI) soup, followed by salmon and broad beans (79 GI), followed by a slice of watermelon (72 GI). Now, while many people would consider this a very healthy lunch, it would draw hoots of derision from low GI fans, who scorn any food that is rated above 70 GI.

However, what they neglect to consider is that each of these foods delivers a very low *quantity* of carbs per serving. A teaspoon of sucrose weighs 4.2g, so that large slice of watermelon contains only a tiny amount more than a teaspoon of (albeit fast-releasing) sugar. Indeed, overall, less than 5 per cent of the total weight of these demonised foods is actually available or burnable carbohydrates. The rest is predominantly water, fibre or protein. So, this rather substantial meal provides a mere 17.6g of carbs. As a result, if you're aiming for 50g per day, you would be bang on target.

By knowing *both* the quantity and the quality of the carbs in your food, you can work out the true effect on your blood sugar. This is called the glycemic load (GL). In essence, GL is simply *quantity × quality*, as the following table shows.

Food	GI	GL	Carbs per serving
Watermelon	72	4.3	4.2g per 120g
Broad beans	79	4.1	5.2g per 80g
Pumpkin	75	4.3	4.3g per 80g
Carrots	92	3.6	3.9g per 80g
	80 (average)	16.3 (total)	17.6g per 360g (4.8%)

As a result, the GL of a particular diet is a far better indicator of whether a person is likely to develop diabetes than either GI or total carb intake alone. Low GL diets are also highly effective at reversing weight gain, diabetes, heart disease and cancer. Indeed, in these respects, they rival the claims of ketogenic diets, but without any need to eliminate a whole food group – carbs. For instance, beans, bread, pasta and rice can all remain on the menu, as long as you remember to have the right *kind* in the right *quantity*. The same is true of fruit, which is usually taboo in low carb diets. Again, though, the amount of a particular fruit you can eat depends on the type of sugar it contains. All of this is taken into account when you calculate the GL (rather than the GI) of any food. You can't cheat with GL.

Anyone who avoids the foods in our sample lunch fails to appreciate that watermelon (4.3 GLs per 120g serving), broad beans (4.1 GLs), carrots (3.6 GLs) and pumpkin (4.3 GLs) all have a low GL, despite their high GI, because they contain small proportions of carbohydrate by weight. Consequently, the total GL score of the meal is a modest 16.3 GLs. In general, to maximise weight loss (and/or regain blood sugar control if you're diabetic), you need to eat a maximum of 40 GLs a day, plus 5 GLs for drinks, so this kind of meal is fine. Later, we'll show you that following such a diet can have a dramatic effect on type 2 diabetes, heart disease and weight loss, with some people able to lose 15lb (7kg) in a month on a 40 GL diet.

Below, we show the radical difference between a low GL and

a high GL diet. The menu on the left is low GL, totalling 40 GLs. If you follow it, you'll feel energised and lose weight. By contrast, the one on the right is a recipe for weight gain and, in due course, diabetes.

Breakfast	GLs	Breakfast	GLs
Bowl of chia porridge	8	Bowl of cornflakes	21
Handful of blueberries	3	Banana	12
Carb-free almond milk	–	Milk	2
Snack		**Snack**	
Punnet of strawberries	5	Mars bar	26
Lunch		**Lunch**	
Substantial tuna salad + 3 oatcakes	10	Tuna salad baguette	15
Snack		**Snack**	
Pear + some peanuts	4	Bag of crisps	11
Dinner		**Dinner**	
Salmon with Kamut bulgur and green beans	10	Pizza with Parmesan cheese and tomato sauce + salad	23
Good Menu Total	40	Bad Menu Total	110

Now, let's look a little closer at ostensibly 'good' low GI foods: that is, foods with a GI score of less than 50 that contain 'slow releasing' sugars. If you ate salmon and white pasta (47 GIs but 10 GLs) with a boiled sweet potato (44 GIs but 13 GLs), followed by a low fat yoghurt (33 GIs but 11 GLs), all washed down with a glass of pineapple juice (46 GIs but 13 GLs), your meal would be very high GL. As a result, your blood sugar and insulin levels would shoot up – a recipe for diabetes – even though you had eaten nothing but low GI foods.

Food	GI	GL	Carbs per serving
Low fat yoghurt	33	11	33g per 200g
Sweet potato	48	13	26g per 150g
White spaghetti	47	10	21g per 180g
Pineapple juice	46	13	25g per 250ml
	43.5 (average)	47 (total)	105g

The sugars in these foods might release slowly, but they all contain *loads* of sugar. The available carbohydrate in this meal is a whopping 105g. That's six times as many carbs as were available in the earlier soup, broad beans and watermelon meal. So, this is still a high carb meal, even though all the foods are 'low GI' and 'slow releasing'.

A food's effect on your blood sugar depends on *both* its GI and the quantity of carbs it contains: that is, its GL. In this example, the total GL score is 47, which is more than you should be aiming for in a whole day! The net effect of eating such a meal on a regular basis would be a massive increase in your blood sugar and a parallel increase in your waistline. Yet, all of the foods have a GI of less than 50. This is precisely why strict adherence to a low GI diet can be detrimental to your health.

Problems with the Low Carb Approach

On the other hand, a similar problem occurs if you take into account nothing but grams of carbs and ignore your food's GI, as most ketogenic diets do.

For dinner, let's say you have salmon and some greens (neither of which contains any carbs) and some Kamut bulgur, which boils like rice but cooks in only eight minutes, followed by a serving of plum crumble (made with three plums, oats, coconut butter and a teaspoon of xylitol). Pretty healthy – right? Yet, only the salmon and greens would feature on most 'low carb' diets, which tend to aim for a maximum of 50g of carbs per day and impose a blanket ban on all 'high carb' fruit juices, fruits and grains. This meal contains 47g of carbs, so you would blow your daily allowance in a single sitting.

Food	GI	GL	Carbs per serving
Kamut bulgur	32	4.5	12g per 25g dry – 75g cup cooked
Oats	50	5	10g per 13g – quarter cup
Plums	29	6	20g per 24g – 3 plums
Xylitol	7	0.5	5g – 1 teaspoon
Total	118	16	47g

However, and this is the crucial point, it's only 16 GL! To lose weight and reverse diabetes, we recommend 10 GL per meal plus 3 × 5 GL for drinks, desserts and snacks – a total of 45 GL per day. So this meal is almost perfect since the 'allowance' is 10 GLs for the meal and 5 GLs for dessert, equalling 15 GLs.

Eamonn, from Dublin, was tired, overweight and depressed. He was also suffering from high blood pressure. So he decided to follow the low GL diet, eating a maximum of 45 GLs per day. 'With the help of the GL diet and exercise I have managed to lose seven stones [44.5kg] in seven months,' he says. 'The way I feel now is completely different. I wake up fresh, looking forward to the day and full of energy. I can't believe how easy it is to follow and I never feel hungry. My blood pressure is normal and I am off all medications. But the most amazing thing is that I'm not hungry.'

If you like to eat cereal in the morning, a substantial bowl of porridge is only 5 GLs, so you can supplement this with 5 GLs of fruit. The illustrations below shows what this means in terms of a variety of fruits.

5 GL of fruit

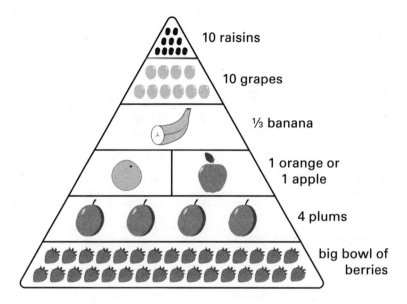

10 raisins

10 grapes

⅓ banana

1 orange or
1 apple

4 plums

big bowl of
berries

As you can see, you can eat loads of berries and plums (which are high in xylose), but not so many apples or oranges (which are high in fructose) and even fewer bananas, dates, raisins and grapes (which are high in glucose).

Similarly, in the low GL diet, dinner comprises half a plate of non-starchy, mainly green vegetables (as in a standard low carb, high fat diet), a quarter of a plate of protein (again, as in a low carb diet) and a quarter of a plate of starchy foods such as rice, potatoes or pasta. This final quarter is the big difference between low GL and ketogenic diets – a fourth of the plate is carbs rather than fat.

As mentioned above, you can allow yourself 10 GLs per meal. The non-starchy veg portion will be roughly 3 GLs and the protein portion 0 GL, which means you have 7 GLs left for the carbs quarter, but what does this mean in real terms? The table overleaf shows you 7 GLs of a variety of foods (both 'good' and 'bad') in terms of both cooked weight and dry weight (the amount you put in the pot).

Food	Cooked weight/amount	Dry weight
Kamut bulgur	190g	60g
Quinoa	120g	40g
Butternut squash		186g
Lentils	175g	70g
Potato (boiled)	2 small	74g
French fries/chips	6–7	47g
Sweet potato	½	61g
Wholewheat pasta	74g	37g
White pasta	66g	22g
Brown rice	70g	35g
White rice	46g	15g

There are photographs of all of these servings at: www.hybriddiet. co.uk/lowGLfoods.

There's a bit more to the low GL diet. In fact, there are three hard and fast rules:

1. No more than 45 GLs per day.

2. Always eat protein *with* carbohydrate.

3. Graze rather than gorge: three meals plus two snacks.

This third rule is another sharp contrast with many ketogenic diets, which advocate no snacks at all, and certainly none with carbs. The assumption with those diets is that you will feel full because of all the protein and fat that you eat during your main meals, so you'll have no need or desire for snacks. Some go even further and advocate two or only one meal per day.

Conversely, the aim of the low GL diet is to ensure that your blood sugar level never falls too low (because that will trigger your appetite) nor too high (because that will trigger insulin release). It achieves this through 'grazing not gorging': in other words, you eat less, but more often. In practical terms, this means breakfast, a mid-morning snack, lunch, a mid-afternoon snack and finally dinner, all with the right low GL carbs as well as protein.

It's easier than you may think. Have another look at the diagram of 5 GL fruit portions on page 69. Any one of these could be eaten as a snack, together with a small handful of nuts or seeds, which are high in protein and fat.

A Spoonful of Sugar (Equivalent)

The message is clear: you must take *both* quality and quantity of carbs into account when planning your diet. Our advice is to eat fewer carbs overall *and* the right kinds.

Dr David Unwin, whom we met in Chapter 2, has found a terrific way to illustrate GL for his diabetic and overweight patients. Instead of trying to explain the concept, he simply shows them the 'teaspoons of sugar equivalent' for each food, as indicated in the table overleaf.

The GI column relates to how quickly or slowly each of these foods releases its sugar. For instance, the GI for strawberries is a relatively low 40 per cent (compared to 100 per cent for glucose). In addition, they have an extremely low glycemic load (just 1 GL), which means that a typical (quite large) 120g portion provides the equivalent of only 0.4g of white sugar. By contrast, while an apple's GI is slightly lower, at 39 per cent, it contains more actual carbs so it has a much higher glycemic load (6 GLs) and therefore it raises blood sugar levels six times as much as the same quantity of strawberries. The last column converts the GL score

Food	GI	Serving size	GL	Teaspoons of sugar
Cereals				
Coco Pops	77	30g	20	7.3
Cornflakes	93	30g	22	8.4
Mini Wheats	59	30g	13	4.4
Shredded Wheat	67	30g	14	4.8
Special K	54	30g	12	4.0
Bran Flakes	74	30g	13	4.8
Porridge	63	150ml	6	2.2
Bread				
White	71	30g	10	3.7
Brown	74	30g	9	3.3
Rye (69% wholegrain rye flour)	78	30g	11	4.0
Wholegrain barley (50% barley)	85	30g	15	5.5
Wholemeal (stoneground flour)	59	30g	7	2.6
Pitta (wholemeal)	56	30g	8	2.9
Oatmeal batch	62	30g	9	3.3
Fruit				
Banana	62	120g	16	5.9
Grapes (black)	59	120g	11	4.0
Apple (Golden Delicious)	39	120g	6	2.2
Watermelon	80	120g	5	1.8
Nectarines	43	120g	4	1.5
Apricots	34	120g	3	1.1
Strawberries	40	120g	1	0.4

Adapted, with permission, from David Unwin's charts in the *Journal of Insulin Resistance* (2016) into the equivalent number of teaspoons of (white) sugar. So, for example, a 120g apple would have the same blood sugar effect as 2.2 teaspoons of sugar.

Part 4 explains how to get the best out of the low GL diet. But does it work? Does eating a slow carb diet really aid weight loss, help to control diabetes, and arrest or even reverse heart disease, cancer and dementia? As the next few chapters explain, yes, it does!

Chapter 8

The Low GL Diet
Reverses Diabetes

An amazing 10 per cent of the NHS's total budget is already spent on diabetes. In the three years since 2015, the number of children and adolescents diagnosed with the condition has risen by 40 per cent. If we continue on this course, the prediction is that over five million people in the UK will be living with diabetes by 2025. This is developing into a major national catastrophe and represents an abysmal failure on the part of the medical establishment.

Yet, the NICE guidelines continue to instruct GPs to 'encourage high-fibre, low GI sources of carbohydrate in the diet'. This is a classic example of a 'quality only' approach: even diabetics are still instructed to eat lots of carbs, as long as they are a little more selective about the *type* they eat. As we have seen, the UK government's 'Eatwell Guide' (see page 13) still recommends a diet that comprises 37 per cent starchy carbohydrates and 39 per cent fruit and vegetables. What it doesn't make clear is that carbohydrates make up over 60 per cent of the calories provided by this diet, while fruit and vegetables only supply 6 per cent of total calories. There is irrefutable evidence that this simply doesn't work for diabetics.

By contrast, two alternative approaches clearly *do* work: the ketogenic (high fat, low carb) diet and the low GL (slow carb) diet. Both deliver a low glycemic load, which tackles the true cause of diabetes at source. The same is true of fasting (intermittent or otherwise) and simply consuming fewer calories. The less food you eat, the less chance there is for your blood sugar and insulin to rise. The question is how low you need to go with your GL in order to get the best result without feeling hungry, which is key to maintaining any kind of diet. Let's examine this in the context of diabetes, before moving on to heart disease and weight loss in the following chapters.

Low GL Equals Low Risk of Diabetes

As we explained in the previous chapter, the best diets take both quality and quantity of carbs into account. In essence, aim to eat fewer carbs overall and more of the right kinds of carbs. The table overleaf shows the progress of 125 of Dr David Unwin's patients who did just that over the course of fifteen months. On average, they achieved a 32 per cent drop in HbA1c (the most accurate long-term measure of blood sugar), a 26.5 per cent drop in tri-glycerides (blood fats), a weight loss of 8.6kg, an 8 per cent drop in total cholesterol coupled with a 13 per cent increase in 'good' cholesterol (HDL), and a 9 (systolic)/8 (diastolic) drop in blood pressure (a decrease of about 7 per cent).[1]

Measure	Start of the trial	After 15 months	Change	Percentage decrease
Weight	96.5kg	87.9kg	−8.6kg	9%
HbA1c mmol/ mol (%)	70.2 (8.6%)	47.9 (6.5%)	−22.3 (2.1%)	32%
Triglycerides	2.23	1.64	−0.69	26.5%
Cholesterol	5.5	5.1	−0.4	8%
HDL cholesterol	1.29	1.46	+0.17	13% (increase)
Triglycerides/ HDL ratio	1.72	1.12	−0.6	35%
Blood pressure	143/86	134/78	−9/8	7%
Gamma GT	87.1	48	−39.1	45%

Norwood Surgery, Southport; used with permission

Thankfully, other GPs are starting to catch on. For instance, the Wokingham Medical Centre recommended a similar low GL, low carb diet to thirty patients with type 2 diabetes and they achieved very similar results after only six months: their HbA1c dropped by an average of 24 per cent and their weight by 9kg, while their levels of triglycerides and cholesterol improved, too.

30 patients	Before	After 6 months	Change	Percentage decrease
Weight (kg)	94	85	9	10%
HbA1c mmol/ mol (%)	63 (7.9%)	48 (6.5%)	15 (1.4%)	24%
Triglycerides	2.3	1.5	0.8	35%
Cholesterol	4.45	5.03	−0.59	–
HDL Cholesterol	1.22	1.65	0.43	35%
Trig/HDL ratio	1.89	0.91	0.43	35%
Blood Pressure	134/80	134/80	0	-

Wokingham Medical Centre; used with permission

The Maidenhead Trial

A medical practice in Maidenhead adopted a more cautious approach. Two of the surgery's patients claimed to have reversed their diabetes after following a low GL diet recommended by a local nutritional therapist – Ann Garry – for three months, so the GPs challenged Ann to test the diet in a larger group comprising twenty-one patients with either diabetes or pre-diabetes and/or significant risk of cardiovascular disease. The criterion for success was set at a 10 per cent drop in HbA1c after twelve weeks, as this is the best long-term indicator of blood sugar control. All of the patients were encouraged to follow the low GL eating plan (see Chapter 23) while also initiating lifestyle changes, such as taking more exercise. Nutritional supplements were not used, as both Ann and the surgery wanted to test the effects of the diet (plus lifestyle changes) alone. All of the clinical markers for chronic disease were measured at the beginning of the programme and after the full twelve weeks, while weight and body composition were tracked throughout the trial.

All of the participants lost weight, with nine losing over a stone (7kg) and one two stones (14kg). The majority also achieved clinically significant reductions in most of the markers.

Measure	Start of the trial	After 15 months	Change	Percentage decrease
Weight	91.8kg	85kg	–6.8kg	7.4%
HbA1c mmol/ mol (%)	51.9 (6.9%)	41.0 (5.9%)	–10.9 (1%)	14.5%
Triglycerides	2.23	1.64	–0.59	27%
Cholesterol	5.27	4.59	–0.68	12.9%
Triglycerides/ HDL ratio	1.47	1.07	–0.4	27%
Blood pressure	137/81	131/73	–4/8	7%

Symons Medical Centre, Maidenhead; used with permission

As the table indicates, the trial easily surpassed the criterion for success, with the patients achieving an average reduction of 14.5 per cent in their HbA1c by the end of the twelve-week trial. However, one of the participants recorded an even more impressive drop – from 7.8 to 5.5 per cent (a 29 per cent decrease). Significant improvements in fasting glucose levels, cholesterol and blood pressure were also recorded by most of the patients.

Henry is a prime example. He weighed 19 stones 2lb at the start of the trial, with an HbA1c measurement of 6.8 and blood pressure of 131/84. After twelve weeks on the low GL diet, he weighed just 16 stones 13lb, his HbA1c was down to 5.8 and his blood pressure was 116/66. Moreover, his cholesterol had declined from 4.2 to 3.7. He says, 'My energy levels were noticeably higher after only a few weeks and the health improvements in both my body and my mind have given me the incentive to maintain these changes for life.'

Such comments were representative of the whole group. Everyone felt they had gained a range of significant benefits from following the programme, including improved energy levels, elevated mood or a lifting of depression, better sleep, less stress and anxiety, and improved confidence and self-esteem. The surgery's GPs and nurses were similarly impressed with the results, and at the time of writing they were discussing the best means of rolling it out throughout the local community.

According to Ann Garry, 'In week one of the programme the patient group appeared defeated, resigned and exhausted, but over subsequent weeks we witnessed a dramatic transformation. They became lively, energetic, engaged and positive, and I'm confident that they are now equipped with the knowledge to continue their journey to optimum health.'

Moreover, it isn't just patients who reap the benefits. Many GPs suffer depression due to the steady decline of their diabetic patients, but it doesn't have to be that way. As David Unwin says, 'Imagine seeing patients who look and feel so much better on a daily basis. These days, I actually look forward to going through the blood test results and seeing positive improvements. How amazing is that?'

The 3-6-36 rule

Another key factor in the success of the trials in Southport, Wokingham and Maidenhead was the encouragement that the participants received along the way. For instance, in Maidenhead, Ann Garry held weekly ninety-minute group sessions with all twenty-one patients. David Unwin's wife, Jen – a psychologist – runs similar groups for his diabetic patients during which she offers advice on what to eat, how to overcome obstacles and the best way to reach their goals.

Psychological research suggests that it takes three weeks to break an old habit, six weeks to make a new habit and thirty-six weeks to hardwire that new habit. Therefore, support group meetings should be held for a minimum of six weeks, with a follow-up session after seven months.

High GL Equals High Risk of Diabetes

Eating a low GL diet isn't just a great way to prevent and reverse diabetes. There is also a direct correlation between a diet's GL and the risk of diabetes. This is important because, if your risk were linked to the amount of calories in your diet (or the amount of fat), then reducing your intake of calories (or fat) would be the way forward. But it isn't as simple as that. Low fat, low calorie diets are neither more predictive of diabetes nor as effective at reversing the condition. Similarly, a diet's GL is more predictive of diabetes than total consumption of carbs.

Four recent studies involving adults without diabetes, adults with pre-diabetes and diabetes, and adolescents illustrate this point. The first, which took place in China, monitored the progress of more than 2,000 middle-aged people and found that those on high GL diets were two and a half times more likely to develop diabetes than those on low GL diets, irrespective of the weight of the participants.[2] The same researchers then looked at the predictability of GL among people who had recently received a diagnosis of diabetes, compared with a non-diabetic group of a similar age. Unsurprisingly, the diabetics had significantly higher GL diets. Moreover, GL was also an excellent predictor of their levels of HbA1c and 'good' (HDL) cholesterol.[3]

The third study, from Argentina, looked at the dietary GL of 273 obese children and adolescents.[4] Obesity increases the risk of falling into metabolic syndrome, which in turn increases the risk of developing diabetes and heart disease later in life. The researchers found a direct correlation between GL and metabolic syndrome, which a quarter of the participants were already exhibiting, despite their young age. Indeed, a high GL diet predicted a fourfold increase in the risk of developing the syndrome as well as low levels of HDL. The final study reported almost identical findings among a cohort of elderly adults: high GL diets were linked to the development of metabolic syndrome, as well as abdominal obesity, high triglycerides, low HDL and high blood pressure.[5] We'll talk more about the importance of increasing HDL and lowering triglycerides in Chapter 10.

All of these studies merely confirmed what we have known for decades: there is a direct correlation between high GL and diabetes. As long ago as 1997, researchers at the Harvard School of Public Health monitored the health of 42,000 middle-aged men[6] and 65,000 middle-aged women[7] over the course of six years. Those who ate high GL diets were one and a half times more likely to develop diabetes than those who ate low GL diets after factors such as age, body mass index (BMI), smoking, physical activity, family history, alcohol consumption and total energy intake were taken into account.

This is such common knowledge among nutritionists that it's almost old hat to say that a low GL diet is better than a low fat diet for controlling diabetes. Indeed, no other conclusion makes sense, given that GL – rather than calories or fat content – is also the best predictor of insulin release. And, as we know, diabetes is all about insulin. While type 1 diabetics have no ability to make insulin and therefore have to inject it, type 2 diabetics have unnaturally high insulin levels because they have become insulin resistant or insensitive. A good illustration of the way in which a diet's GL predicts insulin release was provided by a 2015 study of type 1 diabetics. A group of volunteers were asked to predict their required insulin dose after meals on the basis of either simple number of carbs consumed or GL. Their blood sugar levels were then measured but not disclosed to the participants. Those who predicted their insulin requirements on the basis of GL experienced much more stable blood sugar than the carb counters,[8] which suggests that GL is a much more accurate predictor of insulin release in both type 2 diabetics and non-diabetics. We explain why this is so important in Chapter 13.

In 2004, Dr Maria Pereira, from Brazil's State University of Ceará, designed an ingenious study in which overweight or obese people followed either a low GL diet or a low fat, low calorie diet for two years.[9] After each participant had lost 10 per cent of their body weight, other metrics were used to measure their overall health. This meant that Pereira was able to explore far more than just the obvious benefits of losing weight. She found that those on the low GL diet experienced greater improvements in insulin resistance (blood sugar control), triglycerides (fat circulating in the blood), inflammation and blood pressure than those on the conventional low fat, low calorie diet. The inevitable conclusion was that reducing glycemic load is likely to be more effective in the prevention and/or treatment of cardiovascular disease and diabetes as well as obesity.

The following year, a Canadian study reported almost identical results.[10] Participants who followed a low GL diet for six months not only lost more weight than those on a traditional low fat, low calorie diet but also experienced greater improvements in HDL cholesterol, triglycerides and fasting glucose levels. Moreover, the same pattern was still evident one year after the start of the trial. The researchers concluded that 'implementation of a low GL diet is associated with substantial and sustained improvements in abdominal obesity, cholesterol and blood sugar control'.

This trial confirmed the findings of a Harvard Medical School team who assessed two groups of obese adolescents. The first group followed an unlimited low GL diet, while the second was placed on a standard low calorie, low fat diet. Those on the low GL diet lost more weight and reduced their insulin resistance, while those on the conventional diet became *more* insulin resistant.[11] As we have seen, there is a direct link between insulin resistance and obesity, diabetes and cardiovascular disease.

Generally speaking, if you reduce your carb intake (as you will on either a ketogenic or a low GL diet), you reduce your risk of developing diabetes and other health issues. This is well illustrated by a Harvard School of Public Health study of more than 80,000 women, whose health was monitored over the course of more than twenty years. The conclusion was that low carbohydrate diets are far better than low fat diets at preventing diabetes, especially when vegetable sources provide most of the fat and protein.[12]

By 2011, a total of thirteen rigorous scientific studies had investigated low GL diets. A meta-analysis of the results concluded that people eating very high GL diets had a 20 per cent increased risk of developing type 2 diabetes than those on low GL alternatives.[13] Moreover, GL was found to be a much better predictor of the risk of developing diabetes than GI alone. Further studies have since confirmed these findings. For instance, a 2014 study involving 205,000 participants found that their risk of developing type 2 diabetes was in direct proportion to their dietary GL.[14] Even more alarmingly, those who combined a high GL diet with low intake of cereal fibre (such as oats) increased their risk of developing the condition by 50 per cent! Similarly, researchers who monitored 64,000 Chinese women over the course of four years found that those who ate diets loaded with high GI carbohydrates, primarily in the form of rice, were almost twice as likely to develop type 2 diabetes than those who ate little or no rice.[15]

Can't We All Just Agree that Low GL Makes Sense?

Given the wealth of circumstantial evidence that links high GL diets to heightened risk of diabetes, initiation of metabolic syndrome and worrying increases in all of the markers that signal impending disease, you may be surprised to learn that there have been few large-scale studies into the benefits of a low GL diet. Moreover, researchers have even found it difficult to agree on a universally accepted definition of what constitutes 'low GL'.

This lack of specificity is a big problem throughout nutritional science. For instance, traditional 'low calorie' diets can range between 500 and 1,500 calories a day, while a 'low carb' diet might include just 20g or as much as 150g of carbohydrates. It's like trying to reach a judgement on the performance of all electric cars after testing nothing but a G-Wiz or a Tesla. Even those studies that do specify what they mean by 'low GL' tend to use 100 GL per day as their benchmark, whereas we have found that 45 GL is the optimum level to reverse diabetes.

However, David Unwin doesn't bother to recommend a daily GL figure for his diabetic patients. He just shows them the charts, monitors their blood sugar levels, and gives them their test results, which encourages them to make the right choices after a day or two. It's a refreshingly simple approach!

Chapter 9

Slow Carbs Win for Weight Loss

D ozens of diets have hit the headlines over the last twenty years. Some have advocated eating fewer or virtually no carbs; others have championed slow 'brown' carbs with a low glycemic load over fast 'white' carbs; still others have focused on the benefits of reduced food intake and intermittent fasting, such as eating far less than usual two days a week or nothing at all outside of an eight-hour window each day. Almost invariably, those with the most traction have concentrated on reducing glycemic load through either fewer carbs overall and more slow carbs or simply less food, both of which limit the release of insulin and help the body to maintain an optimum level of blood sugar. These approaches make much more sense than the conventional low fat, low calorie diet, yet many public health bodies, including the NHS, as well as a number of leading diabetes charities and old-school dietitians remain firmly rooted in the past.

Fortunately, though, the tide of public opinion is starting to turn against them, simply because the low fat, low calorie diet does not work. Indeed, there has never been a shred of evidence that it has ever worked over the long term.

Wendy's Story

Wendy is a case in point. Having been overweight her entire life, she was diagnosed with diabetes at the age of forty. She was immediately enrolled in her local NHS weight-loss group, which, of course, extolled the virtues of the low fat, low calorie diet. She also attended a series of clinics that were designed to help her manage her newly diagnosed condition. The instructors told her to steer clear of all fats and to replace the sugar in her tea with sweeteners. Wendy takes up the story:

I knew *that* was wrong. Sweeteners are bad and they could even make me poorly. What to do? I had watched two brothers and my father become seriously ill due to diabetes and I was going down the same road. I felt lost. I'd tried so many different diets and lost a stone or two, only to regain it – plus a few more pounds – every time. Now I was hardly eating at all, yet I was still piling on the pounds. At my heaviest I weighed over nineteen stones (121kg).

My daughter suggested the low GL diet, but past experience warned me that diets make me *gain* weight in the long run, and I didn't want to make things worse. However, I took her advice and gave the low GL diet a trial for one month. I felt sick with worry when I saw the size of the meals. I couldn't finish them because I was so unused to eating proper portions. But my husband, Peter, told me to persevere and give it a month. He even joined me on the diet to give me support.

After the first month, it was time to get weighed and I was shaking and crying with fear. I cried some more when I saw I'd lost a stone, only this time with relief! I could not believe it. I went online and bought Patrick Holford's *Low GL Diet Bible*. I've read that book five times now. Reading it was like coming home. Finally someone knew how I felt. More than that, though, it gave me an answer about how to put it right.

How did I feel after that first month? Well, not exhausted for one thing. My joints did not ache and I realised that, despite my weight, I could run upstairs. My eyesight significantly improved, too, so I felt able to drive again.

I was eating really lovely, tasty meals and feeling full and satisfied. Also, the recipes were excellent because they fitted in with the rest of the family, so no more cooking two different dinners every day.

A year later, I was six stones (38kg) lighter and my HbA1c had dropped from 8.1 to a healthy 5.1. Meanwhile, my waist had reduced from 118cm to 90cm.

I feel fantastic! I am full of life and vitality. No sugar cravings and I can see again! My blood pressure is officially 'textbook' and my cholesterol is just 3.5 – well in the healthy zone. I sleep like a log and wake up an hour earlier than I used to, which means I have gained twelve days of extra time in the last year. Much to my relief, my hair is growing back, too. I have no desire to return to my old way of life.

Of all the diabetics who enrolled in the NHS weight-loss group, Wendy was the only one who didn't regain the weight she lost. In fact, due to her unparalleled success, the group asked if she would star in a promotional video. She gracefully declined, as their low calorie advice had been no help whatsoever!

It's Metabolism, Not Calories, that Really Counts

The idea that 'a calorie is just a calorie', and that the only way to lose weight is to eat fewer of them, is patently wrong. Human metabolism, the bit that stands in the middle of what you put in your mouth and what you weigh, is far too complex. Calorie counting is like saying that one gallon of petrol will always get you exactly forty miles down the road, no matter what car you drive. Yet, hybrid cars routinely deliver 140 miles per gallon, in effect because they have more efficient metabolism than the old gas-guzzlers. How we process sugar and fat depends on numerous factors. For instance, if you become insulin resistant, as Wendy did, those sugar calories convert into body fat much more rapidly. By contrast, if you tune up your metabolism, you can lose weight even if you consume the same number of calories.

Marthinete Slabber, a dietitian, was one of the first researchers to explore this, way back in the 1990s. Fifteen of her volunteers followed a low GL diet for twelve weeks, while fifteen others followed a conventional low fat, low calorie diet. Crucially, the two diets contained identical numbers of calories.[16] The volunteers then switched diets for a further twelve weeks, so everyone got to do both. Both groups lost weight during the first twelve weeks, but those on the low GL diet lost 1.9kg more than those on the conventional diet (9.3kg versus 7.4kg). The second twelve-week period was even more conclusive: those who switched to the low GL diet lost 2.9kg more than those who switched to the conventional diet (7.4kg versus 4.5kg). In addition, fasting insulin levels were significantly lower in the low GL group in both periods – and low insulin is associated with decreased risk of obesity, diabetes and heart disease. This was just the first of several trials, all of which reported similar results.

A decade ago, a meta-analysis of six studies that had looked into the effects of low GL diets on overweight people concluded that these diets are more effective than conventional low calorie diets for weight loss and improving overall health. The researchers declared, 'overweight or obese people lost more weight on a low Glycemic Load diet and had more improvements in lipid profiles than those receiving conventional diets'. The participants on low GL diets – who were assessed over periods ranging from five weeks to six months – also showed much greater improvements in body fat percentage, total cholesterol and 'bad' LDL cholesterol than those on traditional low calorie diets; their 'good' cholesterol (HDL) increased, too. All of these findings suggest that people on low GL diets will enjoy significantly better cardiovascular health than those on low calorie diets while also losing more weight.[17]

Other studies confirmed these results. For instance, six months after the end of the Harvard Medical School trial involving obese teenagers (see Chapter 8), the researchers found the low GL group were still significantly lighter than they had been at the start of the six-month experiment, whereas those who had followed the standard low fat, low calorie diet were now heavier than they had been the previous year.[18] Similarly, in the Canadian study that compared low GL and conventional low calorie diets (see Chapter 8), the low GL group lost an average of 2.8kg while the low calorie group gained an average of 0.2kg. Those in the first group also sustained their weight loss over twelve months.[19]

In 2006, I (Patrick) conducted my own trial and then published the results in the *Journal of Orthomolecular Medicine*. Sixteen volunteers followed my low GL diet for eight weeks, during which time they also took basic supplements (a multivitamin, extra vitamin C and essential omega-3 and -6 fats). The average weight loss was a highly significant 10.25lb (4.65kg) – equivalent to 1.3lb (.59kg) per person per week. Body fat percentage dropped by an average of 2 per cent; all but one of the participants reported greater energy; two-thirds had better concentration, memory or alertness; two-thirds had less indigestion or bloating as well as clearer and less dry skin; and half reported less depression and more stable moods.

There were also significant falls in blood pressure among all of the participants who had hypertension at the start of the trial.[20]

Cut out Fast Carbs to Lose Weight

It's not just the *amount* of carbs that matters. Dr Laura Pawlak has demonstrated that the *type* of carbs is equally important. She fed two groups of rats almost identical diets: same calories, same fat, same protein and same *quantity* of carbs. The only difference was that the first group ate nothing but slow carbs (low GI/GL) while the second group ate only fast carbs (high GI/GL). By the end of the thirty-two-week trial, the low GL rats were 14 per cent lighter and had lost 29 per cent of their body fat, while the high GL group had put on weight.[21]

Another study found very similar results in human volunteers who were placed on one of three diets: low carb, low GL; low carb, high GL; or conventional low fat, high carb. Each diet had exactly the same number of calories and the participants followed them for six months. Those in the low carb, low GL group lost considerably more weight than either the low carb, high GL or the conventional diet group. They also recorded the largest improvements in insulin resistance and the functioning of beta-cells in the pancreas, where insulin is manufactured.[22]

Low Carb or Slow Carb?

So, whether you opt for very low carb in the form of a ketogenic diet (see Part 1) or low GL (low, slow carbs), the end result will be weight loss, if you need it, as well as a much lower risk of diabetes. But is one of these approaches better than the other?

A two-year study explored this question and provided invaluable information on the long-term effects of both diets. The researchers randomly assigned 322 obese people to one of three diets: conventional low fat, low calorie; 'Mediterranean' low calorie (which approximates to our low GL approach); and very low carb, high fat (ketogenic). Weight loss was greatest in the ketogenic group (4.7kg), closely followed by the low GL group (4.4kg), while the conventional group managed only 2.9kg. The first two diets were also more effective in reducing overall cholesterol levels, while diabetics in the low GL group also benefited from significantly lower glucose levels, especially in comparison with those on the conventional diet, who saw their glucose levels increase. So, in conclusion, while the ketogenic approach was marginally better for weight loss and low GL was marginally better for diabetics, both were vast improvements on the conventional low fat, high carb approach.[23]

Tackling the Issue of Rebound Weight Gain

One of the main problems associated with dieting is that the body responds to a low intake of calories by reducing its metabolic rate, which means it burns fewer calories. This is because it thinks it is starving – which, of course, it is, in a way – and does everything it can to conserve the fat you so badly want to shift. As a result, conventional dieters find it increasingly difficult to lose weight even as they eat fewer and fewer calories. An even bigger problem is that they eventually regain any lost weight because they cannot remain on very low calories for ever. They pile on the pounds as soon as their calorie intake increases because their metabolism is still at rock bottom.

The human body's self-regulating and highly complex metabolism is the reason why the 'calories in, calories out' approach never works over the long term. Different foods are metabolised in different ways under different circumstances. It's far more complex than a simple 'calories in from food minus calories out from exercise' equation. Your metabolism is constantly micro-adjusting, so the best health results are achieved when your diet is as 'metabolism friendly' as possible. A low GL diet is just that. For instance, in Maria Pereira's comprehensive, two-year study of overweight or obese adults (see Chapter 8), the participants who followed a conventional low fat, low calorie diet experienced almost a two-fold reduction in metabolic rate compared with those in the low GL group.[24] The conventional view is that you cannot alter your basic metabolic rate, but Pereira's trial proves that you burn more calories while doing nothing on a low GL diet.

Cara Ebbeling and her colleagues at the Children's Hospital in Boston have also reached the conclusion that low GL diets are metabolism friendly.[25] They assigned volunteers to one of three 'maintenance' diets – conventional low fat, low GL diet or ketogenic – in the aftermath of a successful weight-loss programme. Then they monitored the three groups' resting energy expenditure (the number of calories you burn while doing nothing) and total energy expenditure (what you burn doing nothing plus what you burn during physical activity). Those on the low GL and ketogenic diets recorded much greater resting energy expenditure than those on the low fat diet. In other words, the body's metabolism falls less sharply when you eat either low GL or low carb, high fat than it does when you eat low fat. The total calories burned was also greater among those on the low GL and ketogenic diets, with these groups burning up to 300 extra calories each day compared with those on the low fat diet. That's the equivalent of what you would burn in one hour of fairly vigorous exercise. The authors of this important study simply stated that 'a strategy to reduce glycemic load rather than dietary fat may be advantageous for weight-loss maintenance'.

The fact that high fat and slow carb diets have a metabolic advantage (effectively increasing the calories your body burns and improving your ability to burn off excess fat) compared to low fat diets was further demonstrated by a larger and longer trial published in 2018 in the *British Medical Journal*. The trial studied 164 overweight individuals over twenty weeks, who were assigned either a low fat, high carb diet (20 per cent fat, 60 per cent carbs), a moderate fat and carb diet (40 per fat, 40 per cent carbs) or a high fat, low carb diet (60 per cent fat, 20 per cent carbs). The lower the carbs and higher the fat, the more calories they burnt off. The high fat, low carb group burnt off around 300 calories more than the low fat, high carb group, thus proving that a 'calorie is not a calorie'.

The GL of the high fat group's diet was 28 – less than our slow carb phase (45 GLs) and more than our high fat phase (15 GLs). This trial, which cost $12 million should be the final nail in the coffin of conventional calorie theory.[26]

Less Hunger

As well as losing more weight and more body fat, people who follow a low carb diet tend to eat less because they feel much more satisfied after each meal. This was evident in a six-month study of overweight people who were placed on one of three diets, all with the same total number of calories: low carb, all low GI (i.e. low GL); fewer but higher GI carbs; and conventional low fat, high GI carbs.[27] Unsurprisingly, the best results – most weight loss as well as lowest insulin and markers for diabetes – were achieved by the low GL group. However, in addition, the researchers reported, 'Two hours after the breakfast, significantly greater reductions in hunger sensations were shown in subjects allocated to the Low GL diet than in those allocated to the High GI diet.' Maria Pereira's Brazilian study confirmed these findings as the participants on the low GL diet reported significantly less hunger than those on the low fat, low calorie diet.[28]

But why does eating low carb and/or low GL result in less hunger? Researchers at King's College London may have found the answer. They fed volunteers either a high or a low carb meal and then measured the release of a key gut hormone involved in appetite control – glucagon-like peptide 1 (GLP-1).[29] Levels of this hormone increased by 20 per cent among those who had just eaten the low carb meal, so it is hardly surprising that they reported feeling less hungry than the high carb group. More recently, a Chinese study found that a low fat, high carb diet actually *suppresses* GLP-1, which is sure to lead to more hunger.[30] Taken together, these two studies help to explain why a low carb, low GL meal leaves you feeling much fuller than a high carb, high GL meal.

This is an important discovery, as stimulating a natural desire to eat less is obviously a great help to those who want to lose weight. A few years ago, a chef who decided to give the low GL diet a try reported, 'I could just eat and eat and would still be hungry throughout the day. But after two months on the low GL diet I now feel full and can leave food on the plate.' We now know that this is because he's getting a surge of GLP-1 after every meal.

Chapter 10

Slow Carbs and Heart Disease

The simplest and fastest way to reduce your risk of heart disease is to eat slow carbs, avoid sugar and refined carbohydrates, and always combine protein with carbohydrate. This is because too much sugar and refined carbohydrates in your diet raises your glucose levels, which in turn damages your arteries and promotes the release of insulin, which is a major driver of heart disease. Therefore, you should eat fewer carbs, consciously choose those carbs that release their sugar content slowly, and probably eat a bit more protein. By combining protein with carbohydrate (such as porridge with seeds, brown rice with fish, or eggs with oatcakes), you will further reduce the speed at which glucose is released into the bloodstream and thereby lower your glycemic load.

A low GL diet is also an effective way of reducing both blood pressure and LDL cholesterol levels. The level of LDL starts to rise when perfectly normal and healthy cholesterol is damaged by too much glucose and/or oxidants in the bloodstream. This is a widely acknowledged indicator of increased risk of heart disease, but it should be remembered that it is the damaged cholesterol, rather than the cholesterol itself, that causes problems.

As we saw in Chapter 8, researchers at the Harvard School of Public Health monitored the dietary habits and health risks of more than 80,000 women between the 1980s and the early 2000s. One of the most significant findings of this study was that women on a high GL diet were almost twice as likely to develop heart disease than women on a low GL diet.[31] An earlier study involving 75,000 nurses had already reported an almost identical result.[32] The Harvard researchers also found that cardiovascular risk declines further when most of the protein in a diet is derived from vegetable rather than animal sources.

Both of these large-scale, long-term studies clearly indicate that dietary GL is a much better predictor of heart disease than cholesterol level, yet many GPs have not even heard of it, let alone measure it or prescribe low GL diets to reduce cardiovascular risk among their patients.

Blame Carbs, Not Cholesterol

A diet that is rich in carbohydrates, especially sweet foods and those that are made with refined carbs (such as white flour, white rice and sugar), is very bad news for at least five reasons:

1. Your blood sugar peaks several times each day, and the excess glucose will start to damage your arteries, kidneys and healthy cholesterol via glycosylation (see Chapter 4). This damage results in increased levels of LDL cholesterol, which the body's immune system views as an invader and attacks. The resulting 'foam cells' then cause arterial blockages. This is why heart disease and diabetes so often go hand in hand.

2. Your kidney function starts to decline, partly as a result of too much insulin in the bloodstream, which leads to the retention of too much sodium and water, which in turn results in increased blood pressure. This is why kidney failure is so common among diabetics.

3. Damage to the arteries means they are unable to function efficiently, so insulin receptivity declines further while insulin resistance increases.

4. High levels of insulin also inhibit the body's ability to break down fat, so your cholesterol and triglyceride levels start to rise along with your weight.

5. Rebound blood sugar lows will make you tired and trigger the release of adrenal hormones, increasing your stress levels and your blood pressure as your body channels most of its energy into 'fight or flight'. Consequently, it is left with little capacity to heal damaged components, such as blocked arteries.

Nevertheless, the standard medical response to someone who is at risk of developing heart disease is to focus on lowering cholesterol, rather than carbs, which usually means a lifetime course of statins.

A short time ago, I (Patrick) met a middle-aged woman who had recently attended a routine check-up at her local surgery:

> The doctor told me that if my high blood pressure and cholesterol were not reduced within about eight weeks, I would have to go on statins and blood-pressure tablets. But after going to the nurse for six weeks, nothing was happening, so I decided to take control and go on a [low GL] diet. I lost 26lb [11.8kg] within ten weeks. I returned to the doctor, who tested my blood pressure and sent me for a cholesterol test. Both of them were lowered, and the result is that I do not need to go on the statins!

A Low GL Diet Improves Cardiovascular Health: The Evidence

As we have seen throughout this part of the book, countless studies have shown that low GL diets have both immediate and long-term benefits for your health, including lowering total cholesterol and LDL, increasing HDL ('good') cholesterol, stabilising blood glucose levels, improving insulin sensitivity, and reducing the risk of developing cardiovascular disease. It's hard to keep track of all these studies, so let's just pause for a moment and summarise the most significant research over the past twenty years.

- Two groups of overweight or obese people followed either a low GL diet or a low fat, low calorie diet for two years. Those on the low GL diet displayed greater improvements in insulin resistance (blood sugar control), level of triglycerides (fat circulating in the blood), inflammation and blood pressure than those on the conventional low fat, low calorie diet. The researchers concluded that a reduction in glycemic load may aid in the prevention or treatment of obesity, cardiovascular disease and diabetes mellitus.[33]

- One group of volunteers followed a low GL diet while another followed a conventional low fat, low calorie diet. After six months, those on the low GL diet had lost more weight and showed greater improvements in HDL, triglycerides and fasting glucose than those on the conventional low fat, low calorie diet. These health gains were then sustained or enhanced over the next year. The researchers concluded that 'implementation of a low-GL diet is associated with substantial and sustained improvements in abdominal obesity, cholesterol and blood sugar control'.[34]

- Two groups of mice were fed either a low GL or a high GL diet, and their health was monitored. The low GL group ended the experiment leaner with better blood sugar control and lower blood fats than the high GL group.[35]

- A study of 574 adults in Massachusetts between 1994 and 1997 found that higher total intake of carbohydrates, percentage of calories from carbohydrates and glycemic index/ glycemic load were all related to lower levels of HDL and higher blood triglyceride levels. Highly processed carbohydrates had a particularly unfavourable effect on fat profile, increasing cardiovascular risk.[36]

- Participants were assigned to a conventional low fat diet or one of two types of 'Mediterranean' diet. Those in the Mediterranean diet groups received nutritional education plus either free virgin olive oil (1 litre per week) or free nuts (30g per day). Tests were conducted on all three groups after three months. Compared with the low fat diet, the Mediterranean diet produced more beneficial changes in blood sugar levels, blood pressure and HDL. The Mediterranean diet with olive oil reduced levels of the harmful C-reactive protein, which is associated with heart disease. These results show that a Mediterranean-style diet, which is characterised by low GL carbohydrates and increased mono-unsaturated fat intake, is more beneficial to health than a low fat diet.[37]

- Twelve men with type 2 diabetes followed either a low GL or a high GL diet for four weeks. Blood sugar levels after meals were significantly lower among the first group than the second group. Insulin levels and LDL ('bad') cholesterol were also lower in the first group.[38]

- A trial headed by Professor David Jenkins gave two groups reduced calorie diets. The first group ate a small amount of low GI carbohydrates and large amounts of protein and fat from vegetable sources. The second group were given more carbohydrates but less fat and protein. Both groups lost almost 4kg (9lb) in the four-week trial period, but those on the low carb diet experienced greater reductions in their total cholesterol and LDL levels.[39]

- A Chinese study followed 64,000 women with no history of serious illness over the course of twelve years. In that time, 2,991 suffered a stroke, with 609 dying as a result. Dietary GL was the best predictor of both stroke risk and death. (There was no correlation between total carb intake and risk of stroke.) Those on high GL diets were 27 per cent more likely to suffer a stroke than those on lower GL diets.[40]

- The eight-year EPICOR trial in Italy, which involved more than 47,000 people, assessed the significance of diet in cardiovascular risk. Women in the top quarter of GL diets (that is, those who ate the most fast-release sugar and refined foods) had double the risk of heart disease than those in the lowest quarter. There was no equivalent finding among the male participants.[41] However, an almost contemporaneous study in Holland found that men with high GL diets increased their risk of heart disease by 17 per cent, while women increased theirs by 9 per cent.[42]

- A study of over 28,000 Korean men and women found that those whose diets were in the top fifth in terms of GL were three times more likely to have raised levels of coronary artery calcium (CAC), which is a significant risk factor for heart disease as it is associated with hardening of the arteries.[43]

- A meta-analysis of weight-loss studies concluded: 'Overweight or obese people lost more weight on a low-Glycemic diet and had more improvement in lipid [that is, cholesterol and triglyceride] profiles than those receiving conventional [low fat] diets.'[44] Other benefits were more significant reductions in body fat and LDL cholesterol and an increase in HDL cholesterol.

The vast majority of these studies agree that the risk of heart disease declines as the level of HDL cholesterol increases and the level of triglycerides (the form of fat that the body manufactures from sugar and/or alcohol) decreases. So, ideally, you want to see a reduction in your triglyceride/HDL ratio. And the same is true of your levels of LDL cholesterol and blood glucose. (Remember, LDL cholesterol accumulates in the arteries after it is damaged by excess glucose.)

As we saw in Chapter 8, three UK trials placed groups of volunteers on low GL diets, and they all achieved stunning results. In the Maidenhead trial, the participants' triglyceride-HDL ratio dropped by an average of 27 per cent over the course of twelve weeks, while one patient benefited from a 78 per cent improvement. In the Southport trial, there was a 35 per cent drop after fifteen months, with an 87 per cent improvement for one patient.[45] The Wokingham trial did not measure the ratio, but there was a notable fall in the participants' level of triglycerides. All three trials also reported significant decreases in total cholesterol levels, with all of the participants achieving levels that are considered low risk.

Andrew's Story

Andrew, from Dublin, had a cholesterol level of 8.8 mmol/l, so his GP placed him on statins. Six months later, however, his level had fallen to only 8.7. This underwhelming response, plus the unpleasant side effects – including stress and extreme tiredness – convinced Andrew to come off the medication. He needed five coffees a day just to keep going and found it hard to relax in the evening without a couple of drinks. Understandably, he was also gaining weight and not sleeping well.

By chance, it was at this moment that he saw a television programme on which I (Patrick) asked for a volunteer with high
cholesterol to participate in a three-week experiment. He called
the station and I put him on the low GL diet (plus a few supplements). Three weeks later, we met at the TV studio for the 'reveal'.
He had lost 4.5kg (10lb), his energy levels were great, he no longer
felt stressed and he was sleeping much better. Then we tested his
cholesterol: it had dropped to a healthy 4.9!

Keeping your blood sugar balanced not only helps you to lose
weight but gives you more energy and makes you feel less stressed.
By contrast, constant blood sugar peaks and troughs trigger the
body's adrenal hormones, which increase both stress and inflammation. In turn, inflammation leads to heart disease.

Andrew's rapid improvement might sound amazing, but I hear
similar stories all the time.

Eating a Low GL Diet Lowers Your Blood Pressure

High blood pressure is one of the top risk factors for both heart
disease and stroke. A meta-analysis of fourteen trials involving
over a thousand people found that lowering a diet's glycemic
load by 28 GL results in a clinically significant drop in blood
pressure.[46] Yet, millions of people are still given drugs to combat
their hypertension and no advice to cut down on the carbs. Some
are even prescribed two different drugs, and assured that this will
be more effective than taking just one. The trouble is that some of
these drugs are diuretic, so you will pee out many of the body's
vital minerals, including potassium and magnesium, both of
which help to control blood pressure. (Supplementing more than
300mg of magnesium each day is an effective way to lower blood
pressure, as is supplementing more than 500mg of vitamin C.)

David's Story

David was diagnosed with high blood pressure in 1996, when he was just forty-four years of age. His GP informed him that he would have to take beta-blockers, which reduce the impact of adrenalin on the heart, for the rest of his life. Terrified of the potential consequences of ignoring medical advice, at first he dutifully took his recommended dose of beta-blockers, but 'They made it almost impossible for me to exercise. Running felt as if I was carrying a couple of sacks of potatoes.'

After a while, he decided he had to find another way. 'I had a good diet and I exercised, so I wanted to find out why I was having this problem. I bought a blood pressure meter and started to do my own research.' With regular monitoring, he soon discovered that his blood pressure was highly unstable. 'It would be low for a while after I took the drug, but then it would rise out of control. The doctors call this "resistive hypertension".'

David showed his blood pressure readings to a cardiologist who ran a lot of tests and eventually discovered that he had rather high levels of a hormone called aldosterone. As a result, the doctor swapped David's beta-blockers for alpha-blockers, which at least allowed him to start exercising again. But he still didn't feel quite right, so his case was passed on to a professor at a large London teaching hospital. 'He was shocked that my blood pressure was so high and he struggled to treat me for a year, but despite more tests and scans we got nowhere. Eventually, we found that a high potassium diet seemed to help. So I went on a diuretic that con-served potassium and two other drugs. They brought my blood pressure down, and it stayed down.'

However, the idea of remaining on these drugs indefinitely was far from appealing, so, ten years after he was first diagnosed with hypertension, David finally decided to try a low GL diet. The results were rapid and impressive: 'I started feeling giddy within about three weeks, and my monitor showed my blood pressure had dropped right down, so I halved my medication. Two weeks later, the same thing happened again, so I came off the medication completely!' Two months later, David took his latest blood pressure readings to the professor.

David's drop in blood pressure on a low GL diet

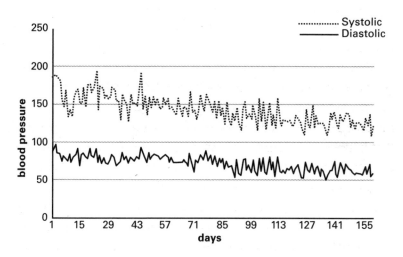

Reproduced with permission

'He was astonished and highly delighted,' remembers David. 'Then I broke the news to him that those figures had been achieved without any medication at all! The initial look of horror on his face changed to total fascination when I explained it was all the result of the low GL diet and that a further benefit was that my cholesterol had dropped from 5.7 to 4.6.'

Thousands of others have also been able to dump the blood pressure tablets simply by switching to low GL.

Chapter 11

The High Carbs Cancer Connection

I n Chapter 3, we saw how cancer cells rely on sugar for their survival because they find it difficult to extract energy from ketones. We also showed that ketogenic diets are recording some staggering results against hard-to-treat cancers, such as brain glioblastomas.

Nevertheless, public health authorities around the world continue to advocate conventional chemotherapy as their main – and often only – treatment for cancer. So, are they ignoring a simple low carb solution that might stem the exponential rise in cancer that has occurred over the last forty years?

The Inexorable Rise of Cancer

Lifetime risk of contracting the disease almost doubled during those four decades and currently stands at one in three. This was also the period when sugar and refined carb consumption increased at its fastest rate in history. Yet, the medical establishment still stubbornly refuses to acknowledge any link between the two, even though everyone – including the World Cancer Research Fund – now agrees that being significantly overweight or obese in adulthood is a major risk factor for at least twelve types of cancer: liver, ovary, prostate, stomach, mouth and throat, bowel, breast (post-menopause), gallbladder, kidney, oesophagus, pancreas and womb.[47] To put the danger into context, being obese puts a woman at almost as great a risk of contracting breast cancer as smoking!

The top five cancers – lung, breast, stomach, colorectal and prostate – were almost unheard of before the twentieth century. Their growth has almost exactly mirrored 'development' – industrialisation, globalisation and cocacolonisation (the spread of US culture around the world). In general, a country's rate of cancer parallels its rise in national income. At the current rate of increase, there will be 24 million new diagnoses of cancer *each year* by 2035. According to the World Cancer Research Fund, the global cost of this epidemic will be an 'astonishing' $458 billion by 2030.

While lung cancer is on the decline as fewer people take up smoking, breast cancer rose by 80 per cent and prostate cancer by an even more startling 350 per cent between 1975 and 2010. Men now have a slightly higher risk of developing the latter than women do of developing the former – roughly one in eight. The incidence of colorectal cancer is expected to increase by more than 100 per cent in those aged between twenty and thirty-four by 2030. That will make it the global number-one killer of people aged under fifty. Indeed, we are already well on the way to that grim statistic: a recent study noted a steady increase in the number of people in Hong Kong contracting this form of cancer before the age of fifty-five. The researchers suggested that obesity was probably the most important cause.[48]

Change Your Diet to Reduce Your Risk

All of this fits neatly with research that consistently links the increased risk of developing cancer to environmental factors, including diet and lifestyle. According to the World Cancer Research Fund, 30 to 50 per cent of all cancers are preventable. by not smoking, changing your diet and keeping physically active.[49] Similarly, the Cancer Research Campaign suggests that four in every ten cancers are preventable.[50]

A decade ago, Dr Walter Willett of the Harvard School of Public Health attributed 14 per cent of all male cancer deaths and 20 per cent of all female cancer deaths to obesity. (By way of comparison, he attributed about 30 per cent of all cancer deaths – male and female – to smoking.)[51] Women who increase from a normal weight at the age of eighteen to overweight or obese between the ages of thirty-five and fifty are 40 per cent more likely to develop breast cancer than women who maintain a healthy weight.[52] Consequently, obesity is now an acknowledged risk factor for developing breast cancer after menopause. The standard explanation for this link is that oestrogens can accumulate in fatty tissue, potentially initiating or accelerating the growth of cancerous cells in the breast. But could it be more to do with eating high carbs – the cause of so much obesity in the first place?

Blood sugar problems are already widely accepted as risk factors for obesity and diabetes, but they are also very accurate predictors of breast cancer. So it's no surprise to learn that diabetics have a heightened risk of contracting cancer. A 2005 review of the previous four decades of research found an 82 per cent increase in the risk of developing pancreatic cancer among diabetics.[53] Around the same time, two Swedish studies reported a 30 per cent increase in the risk of developing colorectal cancer and a 20 per cent increase in the risk of developing breast cancer among those with diabetes.[54]

Ten years later, a group of Italian researchers reported the findings of a study involving almost 50,000 people who were tracked over eleven years. Of the 421 people from the sample group who developed colorectal cancer in that time, most ate very high GL diets. Indeed, such diets roughly doubled the risk of developing this form of cancer.[55] This is consistent with the hypothesis that regular sugar spikes, which trigger insulin release, promote cancer.

Meanwhile, a US study found that high fibre intake – one of the features of low GI and low GL diets – reduces cancer risk, probably because it accelerates gastrointestinal transit.[56] Furthermore, high fibre diets – specifically those that are rich in resistant starch and soluble fibres, such as oats – have the added advantage of feeding good bacteria in the gut, which then produce butyric acid, a kind of fat that nourishes the digestive tract. Without this source of fuel, the gut is likely to become inflamed, which paves the way for colon cancer.[57]

The presence of beta-glucuronidase is another useful indicator of cancer risk, in both the digestive tract and the breast. This carcinogen is made within digestive tracts that are in a state of dysbiosis: that is, they have a deficit of good bacteria, which allows bad bacteria to thrive. It interferes with the liver's ability to break down oestrogen, which results in the hormone's perpetual circulation in the bloodstream and contributes to oestrogen dominance, a known risk factor for breast cancer. Obese people frequently have insufficient butyric acid and large amounts of beta-glucuronidase, as well as far from healthy gut bacteria.

Given that a lack of fibre paves the way for unhealthy changes in the gut, it was no surprise when a group of Chinese researchers concluded that consumption of foods that are rich in fibre protects against breast cancer.[58] Similarly, another study, this time from Uruguay, established a strong link between dietary fibre intake and reduced risk of breast cancer among 700 women.[59] Ten years later, an analysis of pre-menopausal women in the UK found that those with the highest intake of fibre cut their risk of breast cancer in half.[60]

As we saw earlier with the Italian study, eating high GI or high GL foods is associated with increased risk of developing colorectal cancer, and such diets have also been linked with higher rates of breast, pancreatic, ovarian, thyroid, endometrial (womb) and gastric cancer.[61] For example, another group of Italian researchers found that eating sweet foods such as biscuits, brioches, cakes, ice cream, honey and chocolate on a regular basis increased the risk of breast cancer.[62] Conversely, low GI and/or low GL diets seem to reduce the risk of developing breast, colorectal, ovarian and endometrial cancer. Also, survival from all forms of cancers is much higher among those who keep their blood sugar under control.[63]

Another reason why a high GL diet is such bad news is that it increases levels of proteins called 'growth factors', primarily IGF-1, which are major promoters of breast, prostate and colorectal cancer.[64] The excessive insulin that is associated with high GL diets also stimulates the production of hormones, including oestrogens, which are linked to breast cancer. For example, post-menopausal women with high insulin levels have double the standard risk of developing breast cancer.[65]

Does Sugar Cause Cancer?

There is compelling evidence that a high sugar, high GL, high carb diet increases the risk of developing cancer and provides the fuel for cancer cells to grow faster. But could too much sugar – and an increased glycemic load – actually *cause* a normal cell to become cancerous? In other words, is sugar a carcinogen?

Professor Mina Bissell from the University of California, believes that it is: 'A dramatic increase in sugar intake could be a cause of oncogenesis,' she says.

Bissell bases her theory on the fact that a protein called GLUT3 is required to move glucose into cells, and it is found in very high concentrations in cancerous breast tissue. This is yet another example of how cancer cells are magnets for sugar. Bissell's research revealed that pushing up GLUT3 production in healthy cells turned them cancerous, while dampening it down in cancerous cells switched off the cancer-causing genes. The result was that the latter cells became healthy again, even though the cancerous mutations remained.

Nevertheless, all of the major cancer charities still refuse to acknowledge the link between high sugar/high GL diets and cancer. An example of this is Cancer Research UK, who, despite recently promoting obesity as a significant risk factor for cancer, still claim, 'There's no evidence that following a "sugar-free" diet lowers the risk of getting cancer, or boosts the chances of surviving if you are diagnosed.'[66] There is, however, clear evidence that a low GL diet, which effectively means consuming less sugar, does substantially reduce risk.

We can only hope that this current position will change as the medical profession starts to wake up to the fact that what you put in your mouth, especially sugar and fast carbs, has a big influence on cancer risk.

Chapter 12

Slow Carbs Boost Mood and Memory

As we saw in Chapter 6, the brain usually relies on glucose because, unlike the muscles, it cannot burn fat. Ketones are a terrific alternative source of fuel, but the brain has access to them only when the body runs out of glucose and enters ketosis or if they are supplemented in the diet. Therefore, under normal circumstances, the brain needs a constant, consistent supply of glucose to keep it ticking over. So it's no surprise to learn that blood sugar problems – which often culminate in diabetes – are linked to worsening mood and poor memory.

The Brain Bio Centre in London – the outpatient clinic of the Food for the Brain Foundation[67] – has treated thousands of people with mental health issues, ranging from children with ADHD to adults with dementia. The centre always checks for – and usually finds – underlying blood sugar problems. (See Resources at the end of the book for more details on both the Food for the Brain

Foundation and the Brain Bio Centre.) This is because there is ever more evidence that high carb diets push the body into the unhealthy, inflammatory state known as metabolic syndrome, which in turn is linked to ADHD, depression, anxiety, age-related memory decline, dementia and Alzheimer's. Moreover, this process is exacerbated because these diets tend to lack the essential fats and key vitamins that are found in unrefined foods. (See Chapter 19 for more on the role of fats in the brain.)

For instance, one recent trial measured HbA1c and glucose levels in more than 2,000 elderly people over the course of almost seven years.[68] In that time, slightly more than a quarter of the participants developed dementia, and the bottom line was that rising glucose levels were associated with increased risk of developing the condition, irrespective of whether the participants also had diabetes. Non-diabetics who experienced a modest increase in blood sugar levels had an 18 per cent increased risk of dementia, whereas those who already had diabetes at the start of the study or developed it within the trial period had a 40 per cent increased risk.

Other studies have found similar evidence of a link between diabetes and dementia. Back in 2004, researchers at Columbia University stated that people with high insulin levels – the principal hallmark of losing blood sugar control – were twice as likely to develop dementia as those with healthy levels. Moreover, those with the highest insulin levels had the worst memories.[69] The same year, an Italian study also established a link between heightened insulin levels and declining mental function.[70] Similarly, a Puerto Rican study found that people who consumed large amounts of sugar doubled their risk of suffering poor cognitive function,[71] while another US study discovered a strong correlation between blood sugar level and memory loss.[72] Finally, two recent studies – one in Ireland[73] and the other in the United States[74] – established a link between high dietary GL and cognitive decline. Indeed, both of these reports suggested that high GL is even more predictive of the pathological changes associated with Alzheimer's than either high carb or high sugar intake.

While some initial decline in cognitive function is known as 'mild cognitive impairment' (MCI), the next stage is termed 'dementia'. Alzheimer's – which accounts for two-thirds of all cases of dementia – is diagnosed only when a scan reveals shrinkage in certain areas of the brain. One long-term study found evidence that this sort of shrinkage is more common among people with high blood glucose levels, even when those levels are still within what are considered 'normal' (i.e. non-diabetic) limits.[75]

Will Adolescents Develop Dementia?

It's not just adults who are suffering. In just the same way as younger and younger patients are being diagnosed with type 2 diabetes every year, ever more overweight and obese children are experiencing cognitive decline. Although this is not as severe as full-blown dementia, it certainly affects their school performance. Once again, the link to high GL diets seems strong, and the rise in childhood MCI parallels the massive increases in sugar, fructose and sweetened drinks in the Western diet over the past forty years.[76] Up to now, the youngest person to be diagnosed with dementia was just thirty-two years old, but if this trend continues, we may well see adolescents developing the condition in the near future.

Recently, I (Patrick) had a shocking glimpse into that potential future while teaching two groups of sixth-formers in Dubai. On the left sat teenagers from a state school. Out of 1,000 students, 160 already had diabetes. Indeed, many of them were so overweight that they sat across two chairs! On the right were teenagers from a top private school. On the whole, they seemed much leaner and healthier. But what really struck me was that when I asked a question, those on the left stared back blankly. Some were even struggling to stay awake. They were more like zombies than teenagers. By contrast, those on the right could engage, think and respond. This kind of attention deficit is not going to be helped by drugs. All of these kids should be on a strict low carb diet, which will give them more energy, improve their concentration and quite possibly reverse their diabetes.

Sugar Shrinks Your Brain

One of the effects of the high carbohydrate, sugary diet these teenagers are likely to be eating is that it raises the amount of glucose in their blood, along with the hormone insulin. Research shows that having high blood glucose for a long time can shrink an area of the brain known as the hippocampus, which is involved in laying down memories. Too much insulin and glucose can also crank up the body's main energy controller, mTOR, and a number of animal studies have found that it's also linked to brain shrinkage and cognitive problems.[77] There is also clear evidence of mTOR's involvement in the brain shrinkage that affects Alzheimer's.[78]

Sugar Makes You Angry

You may be furious that the food industry, governments, doctors and health officials have all allowed the situation to reach this stage. However, part of your anger may be attributable to a high sugar, high GL diet, which researchers have found increases aggression and even contributes to criminal behaviour. For instance, a ground-breaking study in the *British Journal of Psychiatry* discovered that excessive consumption of confectionery at the age of ten is strongly associated with convictions for violence in adulthood.[79] Similarly, in Finland, Dr Matti Virkkunen discovered that every single one of a sample group of sixty-nine habitual offenders had blood sugar problems.[80]

The good news is that a low carb diet provides an almost immediate remedy. When 1,382 detained juvenile offenders were placed on a reduced sugar diet, there was a 44 per cent reduction in their antisocial behaviour.[81]

But it's not only offenders who suffer as a result of unhealthy diets. A study of eighty A-level students in the West Midlands found that skipping breakfast was associated with a 30 per cent shorter attention span.[82] Similarly, when 133 US elementary school students attended a breakfast programme for four months, their maths grades increased and their rates of absenteeism and lateness both decreased.[83]

Once again, the most important aspect of a child's diet seems to be GL. Researchers in Washington found that the cognitive performance of eighty-three hyperactive eight to thirteen-year-olds declined significantly when they ate a high GL breakfast (two slices of buttered white toast) rather than a low GL breakfast.[84] High sugar, high GL diets have also been linked to social withdrawal, anxiety, depression, delinquency and aggression.[85] One study of dyslexic children even found that a high sugar diet caused more erratic eye movements than a sugar-free diet.[86]

Sugary sweets may be the universal currency for treats, but what sort of treat is it to give a child this sort of start in life? A wise parent and child would say, 'No sugar thanks, I'm sweet enough already!'

The Cognitive Function Test

One of the many problems with cognitive decline is that sufferers are often unaware that it is happening. Also, since the brain shrinks irreversibly as Alzheimer's develops, it's vital to find out sooner rather than later. That's why we offer a simple, accurate and free online Cognitive Function Test at www.foodforthebrain. org. It takes only twenty minutes and helps to identify which diet and lifestyle changes are likely to make the biggest difference for you. To date, over 300,000 people have taken this test.

Part 3

Dual Fuel Advantages

Variation, not moderation, is the key to health. We are evolutionarily designed to oscillate between periods of relative 'feast' and 'famine', which sets up a healthy cycle of growth and repair. This is achieved by switching from a slow carb diet to a high fat diet, supported by intermittent fasting. In this part you will learn why variation is the key to disease prevention and why it's important to initiate ketogenesis every now and again by eating a high fat diet, or fasting, or a combination of the two. We will also show you how to break free from carb cravings and addiction.

Chapter 13

Meet Your Lean, Mean Energy Machine

Human cells are microscopic specks, no more than 10 micro-metres across (one 100,000th of a metre), but each is an industrial estate packed with various units, all of which are vital for its survival. Some of these are familiar, such as the repository of genetic information that is held in the central nucleus, or the nearby protein-making factory (ribosome) that gets its manufacturing blueprints from our genes. Dotted around are thousands of power plants (mitochondria) that generate all of the energy we need to function.

Like all industrial units, each cell must have a reliable supply of fuel, ways of balancing internal demand with available supply, a dedicated system for transporting the fuel to the various units and a reliable back-up system to deal with any power cuts.

It may function on a micro-scale, but the complexity of a cell's energy system is breathtaking. You might assume that we already have a good understanding of something as basic and essential as how the body and brain generate and use energy. But even as you read this, researchers are uncovering ever more of the ways in which the body converts what we eat into fuel and then routes it along the paths of least resistance.

As we saw in Part 1, your muscles and organs, including your brain, can run quite happily on either ketones, which are derived from fat, or glucose, which is derived from carbs. Both end up delivering ATP – the packets of energy on which all of the body's cells rely. In addition, the muscles (but not the brain) may derive energy from a type of fat known as triglyceride, which is shaped like a capital 'E', with a backbone of glycerol (a form of glucose) and three horizontal bars of fatty acids. The liver can also transform the amino acids in protein into glucose when the latter is in short supply. This usually involves breaking down some of the body's own muscles because these are the most readily available sources of protein, which is one reason why you will lose muscle mass if you fast for too long and why people on a ketogenic diet need to ensure that they eat a sufficient amount of protein.

All of these fuels are routed to the cells' mitochondrial power plants, where they are fed into a remarkably efficient 'electron transport system' that generates the vast majority of our ATP power. This system is totally dependent on a steady supply of oxygen, but we can also generate a limited amount of energy from stored glucose in the absence of oxygen in a process known as glycolysis (otherwise known as anaerobic – 'without oxygen' – metabolism). You rely on this when you sprint, because you can't breathe enough oxygen to meet your body's energy demands in the normal way. Glycolysis is also used by cancer cells to fuel their rapid growth.

How your body generates energy

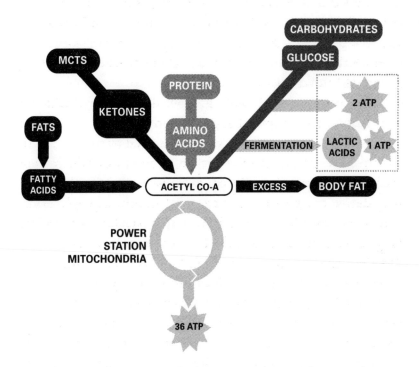

Lactic acid, which is usually demonised as a 'toxic' waste product that makes your muscles tight, is produced during glycolysis. However, the human body is so efficient that it manages to squeeze another drop of energy out of it. Lactic acid is also created during fermentation, so you eat it whenever you have sauerkraut or natural yoghurt. Finally, a very hot topic right now is whether MCT oils – which the liver turns into ketones – might also power the brain via the so-called 'astrocyte–neuron lactate shuttle', using lactic acid as fuel.[1]

With so many energy-generating options available, you would think we'd all be leaping about, full of vigour. However, our modern Western diet is throwing a spanner into this highly effi-cient system, channelling excess, potentially energy-generating food into redundant body fat, and leaving us exhausted, both physically and mentally.

To understand why this happens, and why it is the key to almost every major chronic disease, we need to introduce two main characters: insulin and mTOR. Both of these are essential for good health. However, when they start to spiral out of control, they can send you hurtling down the path of illness and weight gain.

The Insulin Balancing Act

The big problem with conventional approaches to diet is the ill-founded belief that calories in (from diet) minus calories out (from exercise and the energy needed to run your body systems, i.e. your metabolism) is the only thing that determines your weight. While it is true that you would grow if you did nothing but eat, and you would shrink if you did nothing but exercise, this ignores all the metabolic complexity, and flexibility, that is built into our design. In part, that flexibility is controlled by the hormone insulin.

This is why Harvard Medical School's Professor of Nutrition, David Ludwig, puts insulin at the heart of his 'Carbohydrate–Insulin Model of Obesity', which really should replace the outdated 'calories in, calories out' approach. Put simply, the conventional recommendation to eat low calorie by cutting fat because it has the most calories per gram (1g fat = 9 calories while 1g protein or carbs = 4 calories) means you end up eating lots of carbs, which means more insulin production, which means more sugar is converted into fat and stored in the body. Furthermore, as the insulin drives down your blood sugar, you start to feel hungry.

Why ketogenic and low GL diets work, while low fat, high carb diets fail

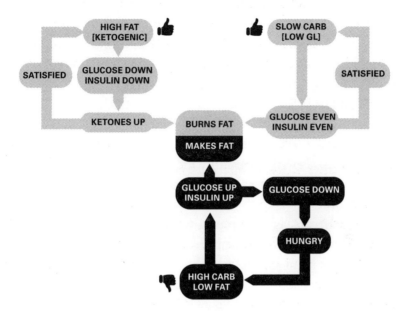

If you eat the opposite – a high fat, low carb diet – your insulin level falls, which drives fat *out* of storage to meet the body's energy requirements. Furthermore, the fat satisfies your hunger. Alternatively, if you eat low, slow carbs – that is, small amounts of slow-releasing carbohydrates – your body doesn't need to produce much insulin, so no fat is stored and you don't suffer the blood sugar dips that drive hunger. The Hybrid Diet incorporates both of these options.

Insulin isn't 'bad' per se. It's an essential growth hormone. However, too much of it, and specifically developing the condition known as 'insulin resistance', lies at the heart of almost all of today's endemic non-infectious diseases. Insulin resistance is a bit like an addiction: your body keeps needing more and more to have the same effect. This leads to very high blood levels (hyperinsulemia), which has all sorts of damaging effects.

mTOR – the Body's Fat Controller

Another energy tsar works alongside insulin: mammalian target of rapamycin – or mTOR for short. (Rapamycin is an immuno-suppressant, so the name is a reference to the enzyme it inhibits.) mTor is a sort of general contractor that is in charge of the major repair projects that your body is constantly undergoing. As Professor David Sabatini, biologist at the Massachusetts Institute of Technology, who studies the basic mechanisms that regulate growth, says '[mTOR] has a finger in every process in a cell'[2]. For instance, as well as carefully monitoring amino acids in the body and proteins in the diet, it responds to and organises signals from insulin.

The details are very complicated, but the bottom line is simple. Ultimately, mTOR is a prudent chancellor that runs your internal economy. Its main job is to promote growth, so it has to monitor the body's fuel supplies closely. If they start to run low, either mTOR switches itself off or it is switched off by 'autophagy', which assumes responsibility for repair and restoration while the body waits for fresh supplies. A ketogenic diet and/or intermittent fast-ing can turn on this cellular clean-up mechanism (see Chapter 14). Then, if you choose to the follow the Hybrid Diet, you will reactivate mTOR when you shift back to slow carbs.

Unfortunately, this highly sophisticated, efficient system, which has been honed by millions of years of evolution, has been caught out by the massive oversupply of carbohydrates in the modern world, and the associated exponential increase in blood glucose levels.

The ketogenic diet became popular because it promised a healthy alternative to overdosing on carbohydrates and achieved rapid, impressive results in terms of both weight loss and revers-ing diabetes. These are the natural consequences of a high fat diet because the body releases much lower quantities of hormones such as insulin and IGF-1 (insulin-like growth factor) – both of which are linked to weight gain – and, crucially, turns off mTOR altogether.

Unsurprisingly, a new narrative quickly emerged in which mTOR was blamed for the obesity epidemic, diabetes and much more besides. The theory went that, while we need it to grow during childhood, by the time we arrive in middle age the growth it promotes is more likely to be cancerous, a bulging waistline or a build-up of plaque in the brain. As a result, the notion took hold that the secret to living a longer, healthier life is to turn off mTOR *permanently*. In short, it became public enemy number one – the new saturated fat or cholesterol – and pharma companies rushed to develop drugs that would block it, then marketed them as anti-ageing treatments. However, this is not such a great idea, as the first drug to do just that, the one that gave mTOR its name – rapamycin – is associated with insulin resistance and sky-high levels of blood glucose when it is used in the treatment of cancer. Indeed, anywhere between 13 and 50 per cent of patients who are treated with rapamycin develop diabetes.[3]

Moreover, the vilification of mTOR was based on a misunderstanding of how it works. Our bodies and specifically the mTOR network developed at a time when the human race had to survive through alternating periods of food shortage and plenty, due to the variable seasons and harvests. So we are designed to switch seamlessly between the two, and the Hybrid Diet allows us to do just that.

Your body is in growth mode when mTOR is switched on, but that doesn't mean that you just pile on ever more pounds of fat. For instance, it is activated by and works with insulin and IGF-1 to build up muscle. This is crucial, because maintaining muscle tone is vital for health, especially as we get older. mTOR activation is also essential for the cell division that we need to replace exhausted blood cells and worn-out gut lining. It is thanks to mTOR that we are able make 2,000 new white blood cells every second and replace our gut lining, which is the size of a tennis court, every four days.

mTOR is switched off at the start of exercise in order to maximise the delivery of fuel to the muscles. However, it is reactivated as soon as you stop in order that your body can resume its routine repair tasks and start to lay down more muscle, if necessary. This is why you should always eat protein after exercise if you want to build or maintain muscle. (By contrast, coffee suppresses mTOR, so make sure you drink it before exercising, rather than afterwards.) Different types of exercise affect mTOR in different ways, as you will see in Chapter 15, where we also explain why intermittent fasting has health benefits precisely because of its effects on insulin and mTOR.

Finally, you will find it very difficult to fight off an infection if you permanently deactivate mTOR. This is because it plays a crucial role in the immune system's rapid production of T cells during glycolysis. The downside is that cancers' rate of growth also increases during glycolysis.

Nutritional Yoga

By switching between a high fat phase – which turns off mTOR and growth, and turns on autophagy – and a slow carb phase – which promotes healthy growth and repair – you get the best of both worlds and allow insulin, IGF-1 and mTOR to orchestrate all of the growth processes you need to thrive.

One of the interesting effects of taking a break from slow carbs and running on ketones for a while is that you will have even better blood sugar control when you return to the low GL diet. This is because your metabolism gains flexibility in the ketogenic phase and you become 'carb adapted' – able to use carbs more intelligently. Moreover, after some time on the low GL diet, you will be 'fat adapted' when you choose to switch back to the ketogenic diet. This means that you will enter ketosis more rapidly, and the symptoms of 'keto flu' (see page 46) will be milder.

This increased metabolic flexibility is due in part to reversing insulin resistance and becoming more sensitive to the hormone's effects, but it is also linked to the fact that mTOR is being turned on and off appropriately. This means that your body learns how to keep blood sugar low, and weight and energy levels balanced. Also, by experimenting with the two principal fuels – glucose and ketones – and monitoring their effects (see Chapter 26), you will become much more aware of the impact of specific foods and drinks, which will help you to make better choices.

Think of it as a form of nutritional yoga in which you use all of your energy-generating options to keep yourself flexible and well adapted.

Why Dual Fuel Has Become a Problem

As we have seen, the fact that our bodies can run on either glucose or ketones gave us a huge evolutionary advantage because we could wolf down abundant carbs in the summer and survive through the winter on our reserves of fat. However, many people's diets are very different now, and this has contributed to the rise of many of the chronic diseases of the twenty-first century. Year round, people gravitate towards junk food that is almost exactly 50 per cent sugar and 50 per cent fat – a malign 'sweet spot' that is virtually unknown in nature, as the following list indicates:

- Grains are mostly carbs and a little protein.

- Beans are mostly protein and a little carbs.

- Nuts and seeds are mostly fat and protein.

- Meat, fish and eggs are fat and protein.

- Fruit is almost all carbs.

- Hard cheese is fat and protein.

- Milk is fat (49 per cent), protein (21 per cent) and carbs (30 per cent).

A neuropharmacologist named Paul Kenny discovered this preference for the fat–carbs combination when he fed rats a variety of different diets.[4] First, he offered unlimited amounts of sugary foods to one group and unlimited amounts of fatty foods to another. Amazingly, both groups were able to control their intake, and it was over a month before either gained any weight. However, when Kenny offered them half-fat, half-sugar food – such as you would find in a cheesecake – the rats would 'dive head first into a slice and gorge so vigorously that it covers their fur in blobs. It's not pleasant.' Moreover, after this initial binge, the rats would continue to graze, returning to the food time and again, as if the internal off switch that should have told them they were full had malfunctioned. They also stopped exercising and gained significant weight in the first week of the experiment. They were even prepared to subject themselves to a mild electric shock in order to get to the junk food. Finally, when Kenny tried to reintroduce a healthier diet, the rats went on hunger strike and refused to eat it!

Foods that Trigger the Body's Fat-Storing Hormones

Fortunately, as we have seen, we can overcome this sort of junk-food addiction by adopting a ketogenic diet. As yet, though, we haven't explained why our version of this diet doesn't result in more body fat.

First, let's be clear: eating nothing but large amounts of fat will lead to some weight gain. While such a diet won't trigger immediate insulin release, it will stimulate the release of two other fat-storing hormones: GIP (glucose-dependent insulinotrophic peptide) and ASP (aceylation stimulating protein). However, these two hormones will promote only modest storage of excess fat as long as your blood sugar remains low. The problem comes when you combine large amounts of fat with large amounts of carbs, because carbs trigger the release of insulin, and insulin boosts the production of ASP. Moreover, ASP then returns the favour by stimulating the release of even more insulin! It's a vicious cycle that you should try to avoid at all costs

Also, although fat on its own is not particularly satisfying, a combination of fat and protein is (and the same is true of ketones). Similarly, eating carbs with protein slows down the carbs' release of glucose, thus lowering the meal's glycemic load. Therefore, a good supply of protein is an essential part of the Hybrid Diet.

Interestingly, protein actually stimulates the release of insulin, but it also promotes the secretion of another hormone – glucagon – which raises the amount of glucose and fatty acids in the blood, thereby effectively cancelling out the effect of the insulin. So, while eating nothing but protein does not make you fat, it's not good for you. You can make a little glucose from the amino acids, but not nearly enough to meet all your needs. As a result, you will still crave carbs whenever your blood sugar dips.

The consequences of eating carbs, fat and protein – and various combinations of the three – are summarised in the table below.

Food	Insulin level	Glucagon	Hunger	Fat storage
Carbs and fat	+++++	No change	++++++	++++++
Carbs only	++++	No change	++++	++++
High GL carbs and protein	++++++	++	+++	++++
Low GL carbs and protein	+++	++	+	
Fat and protein	++	++	+	

As the table indicates, the best way to pile on loads of weight is to combine lots of fat with lots of sugar, because your bloodstream will be flooded with the fat-storing hormones GIP and ASP as well as insulin, which not only promotes fat storage itself but also stimulates the release of more ASP. The end results are high levels of blood sugar and poor appetite control, so you will eat more than you need and become a fat-storing machine.

This is why the modern Western diet is such bad news, and why Paul Kenny's rats were prepared to suffer electric shocks to get their junk-food fix. Is it any wonder that so many weight-watching programmes have virtually no effect? They are the equivalent of offering an alcoholic a glass of water! Fortunately, as Chapter 16 explains, there is a better way to kick the habit.

Why Dairy is Not the Answer

Dairy products, such as cheese, are not closely associated with significant weight gain and they also deliver the fat–protein combination that is so conducive to good health. However, we still believe that they should be eaten sparingly. This is because milk – whether human or cow's – is the only food in nature that mirrors the high carbs/high fat composition of junk food (see page 128), on account of the fact that it is specifically designed to maximise weight gain in new-born infants. True, it also contains protein, but it still triggers the release of three to four times as much insulin as you would expect, given its glycemic load.[5] Moreover, milk contains casomorphin – an addictive opioid.[6] This is another miracle of evolution because it encourages babies to breastfeed and build up vital reserves of fat.[7] But that addictive quality makes dairy products a recipe for weight gain in adults, too, especially when combined with sugar and carbs, as shown in Paul Kenny's cheesecake-addicted rats.

Many low carb diets are heavily reliant on dairy – especially those foodstuffs that contain the least carbs, such as butter, ghee, various cheeses and fully fermented yoghurts (the bacteria turn milk sugar – lactose – into lactic acid) – and it is not our intention to demonise it here. Indeed, some dairy might be advisable if you are in the high fat, ketogenic phase of the Hybrid Diet because it reactivates mTOR, which will improve your immune system's responsiveness and enable your body to undertake essential muscle repairs. However, over-reliance on dairy products is a bad idea because they can stimulate mTOR- and insulin-related growth signals,[8] which could encourage the growth of cancerous cells. See page 213 for more on this and some excellent non-dairy alternatives.

Finally, milk is not an essential or an evolutionarily consistent food for adults. No other mammals consume it beyond the early, rapid-growth phase of life, and nor did we until relatively recently. Our hunter-gatherer ancestors certainly didn't spend their time milking buffaloes and making cheese. They got all the protein they needed from other sources.

Chapter 14

Switching on Autophagy: The Cellular Clean-up

Manufacturing and energy generation create as much waste and junk on the nano-scale, within cells, as they do on the macro-scale, in our global environment. Therefore, an efficient rubbish-removal system for each of our billions of cells is essential if our bodies are to continue functioning properly.

The one we have – which is known as autophagy (literally 'self-eating') – not only hoovers up dead and damaged proteins but also disposes of much larger units, including burned-out mitochondria. All this waste matter is then tipped into a pit that is brimming with enzymes, where much of it is recycled into fresh energy supplies and the raw materials to create new proteins.

When you start a ketogenic diet, the sharp drop in carbohydrates immediately triggers the starvation response. As the levels of glucose and insulin in the blood start to decline, the body's mTOR network – which promotes cell growth when supplies of glucose are high (see Chapter 13) – switches off and autophagy redoubles its collection and recycling efforts. These are just two of the mechanisms that are involved in losing or gaining weight, sending fuel around the body and growing new cells. Crucially, they cannot function simultaneously: when the mTOR network starts, autophagy stops, and vice versa. Understanding how the whole system works will give you a better chance of making it work well for you.

How autophagy works

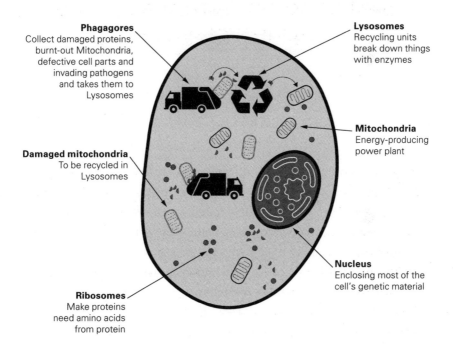

Phagagores
Collect damaged proteins, burnt-out Mitochondria, defective cell parts and invading pathogens and takes them to Lysosomes

Lysosomes
Recycling units break down things with enzymes

Mitochondria
Energy-producing power plant

Damaged mitochondria
To be recycled in Lysosomes

Nucleus
Enclosing most of the cell's genetic material

Ribosomes
Make proteins need amino acids from protein

Millions of microscopic bin lorries called phagophores collect the accumulated rubbish. These ever-expanding trucks trundle around the body's cells, engulfing dead or damaged proteins, bacteria, viruses and exhausted mitochondria as they go. Next, they transport all of the waste products and foreign bodies they have collected to the lysosome – a large bubble filled with enzymes that dissolve proteins into their constituent amino acids. These can become a valuable extra source of fuel for the mitochondria or provide the raw materials for new proteins, which are manufactured in the cells' ribosomes. However, if the body continues to starve – and energy remains in short supply – the ribosomes themselves may be broken down into their component amino acids to provide some emergency fuel for the mitochondria. When the crisis is over – either because glucose supplies have been restored or ketones are now available – growth resumes and the recycled amino acids are once again turned into new proteins.

Autophagy's crucial role in keeping the body supplied with fuel is sometimes evident right at the beginning of life. If the supply of food from the mother stops for any reason, the baby is able to function perfectly well – for a time – on amino acids produced during autophagy. Then, later in childhood, autophagy alternates with mTOR activation to ensure that the growth process proceeds smoothly.

However, once we are fully grown, the body benefits from spending more time in the autophagy (clean-up) phase and less time in the mTOR (growth) phase. One of the best ways to achieve this is simply to eat less, possibly by going on a calorie-controlled diet. As early as the 1930s, it was discovered that animals that are fed 30 per cent less than normal are very healthy with good metabolic markers, such as low blood pressure, low glucose and insulin, and a healthy body mass index.

Moreover, in addition to providing emergency energy supplies, autophagy seems to offer some protection against brain disorders, including Parkinson's disease. Neurons use a lot more energy than other cells, so the brain's mitochondria need to be especially efficient. However, as we age, the mitochondria's system for mopping up the oxidants that are released during energy production starts to deteriorate and DNA can be damaged as a result. Fortunately, though, as we have seen, autophagy weeds out the worst mitochondria before they can do too much harm. This is just one of the reasons why it's so important to kickstart the repair process on a regular basis.[9]

Another is that cancerous cells find it harder to multiply and spread during autophagy. This is because phagophores quickly identify the defective cells, hoover them up, and deposit them in the lysosome, where they are broken down. In addition, 'Autophagy limits oxidative stress, chronic tissue damage, and oncogenic [cancer cell] signalling, which suppresses cancer initiation.'[10] Unfortunately, if a tumour is given the chance to establish itself, the balance of power may shift, as it will be able to use the amino acids that are produced during autophagy as fuel to meet its very high energy demands and expand into surrounding territory.[11]

It's possible that inadequate or malfunctioning autophagy is also a factor in the development of Alzheimer's, given that the condition is characterised by a build-up of plaque and other waste products in the brain.[12] Indeed, recent research suggests that a wide range of illnesses may be linked to damaged mitochondria that have lost the ability to burn fat or glucose efficiently.[13] A case in point is chronic fatigue syndrome, in which energy production is obviously compromised.[14] As such, it is imperative to keep clearing out the worst-performing mitochondria through autophagy.

However, autophagy itself tends to become less efficient as we get older, probably because the body's lysosomes lose some of their ability to recycle amino acids. The ketogenic diet – and/or fasting – might provide the answer because it pushes the body into autophagy on a much more regular basis and therefore forces the lysosomes to keep working. This is one reason why the approach has been proposed as a treatment for chronic fatigue syndrome.[15]

The pharmaceutical industry and medical researchers are currently exploring ways to improve lysosomes' performance through genetic engineering and developing ever more powerful drugs to block mTOR. However, we believe that the Hybrid Diet is a much more natural way to achieve the same goals. As you switch from a high fat to a slow carb diet, then back again, your system cycles through predictable, controllable periods of growth (more cells, more muscle mass, more troops for your immune system) and periods of clean-up and repair (when autophagy is the key player).

It's what we have evolved to do.

Chapter 15

The Value of Intermittent Fasting and Exercise

Although we have concentrated on the high fat route to ketogenesis, there is another way: simply not eating.

Dieting – or more precisely fasting – used to mean getting into a boxing ring with your body and going as many rounds with hunger as you could before throwing in the towel. However, the ketogenic diet changed all that by pulling a fast one on hunger and knocking it out with fat. You get all of the well-known benefits of fasting while keeping hunger at bay. This has proved a boon to diabetics and others who want to lose weight and reverse the symptoms of metabolic syndrome. Moreover, it has allowed a range of obscure biochemical players in our metabolic engine rooms – IGF-1, mTOR and autophagy, among others – to receive the attention they deserve (see Chapters 13 and 14).

Our ever-increasing knowledge of these chemicals and processes has transformed our attitude to fasting. While it has long been a staple of countless medical and religious traditions, it had become a 'no pain, no gain' practice to be endured rather than enjoyed, like cold baths. Now, though, because we understand *why* it is so beneficial, we can view it as a rewarding part of a healthy lifestyle.

Why IF?

Periodic fasting is so advantageous because it turns off some processes that cause excessive weight gain and inflammation, and turns on others that dispose of accumulated junk and carry out essential repairs. A quick and easy way to reap the bene- fits – which include weight loss, less cell damage due to harmful oxidants and a tune-up of the immune system – is to choose one of the many intermittent fasting (IF) options. These generally involve eating about half as much as usual for one or two days a week, or nothing at all for shorter periods of time.

The best known of the first type of IF is the so-called '5:2 diet': two days on 500 to 600 calories and the rest of the week eating whatever you want. A recent study of diabetics compared this option with eating 1,200 to 1,500 calories every day. The weight loss was almost identical on the two diets, so the conclusion was that IF is 'an effective alternative for diabetics'.[16] However, the researchers neglected to mention that you lose less muscle mass during IF than you do during daily calorie restriction,[17] so per- haps the former should be considered as preferable to the latter, rather than merely an alternative. 'On a regular weight loss diet, we would expect to see a loss of 75% fat and 25% muscle,' writes Krista Varady, Associate Professor of Kinesiology and Nutrition at the University of Illinois, Chicago. 'But on IF the loss is 90% fat and 10% muscle.'

The other common type of IF involves either reducing your cal- orific intake or eating no calories at all for various lengths of time in each twenty-four-hour period. A common starting point is to use the seven or eight hours we spend asleep as part of the fasting period. This is known as the '16:8 diet' if you eat nothing from, say, 10 p.m. in the evening until 2 p.m. the following afternoon.

A Few Words of Caution

There are still plenty of unanswered questions about IF diets. They are certainly popular, and many people find them relatively easy to follow, but few have been subjected to rigorous scientific trials and many probably never will be because of the huge number of variables, such as different timings, preceding and subsequent dietary regimes, and how many days a week are involved.

Advice on what may be consumed during a 'no-calorie' IF day also varies widely. Typical options are lemon juice, tea, black coffee and maybe a small portion of bone broth or kombucha, as long as you stay under about 50 calories. Other IF diets advocate the addition of various supplements.

Reports of dangerous side effects are very rare, but certain groups are advised not to fast either intermittently or otherwise, including women who are pregnant, trying to conceive or breast-feeding and anyone with a history of eating disorders.

There are also practical considerations. Most of us prefer to eat quite late dinners – often after putting the children to bed or working late – so starting the fasting period relatively late in the evening makes sense for many people. However, a number of small studies have found that participants who shift from eating late to no later than 6 p.m. lose an average of an extra 7lb on an identical diet. This suggests that the best option is to follow an IF diet that also rules out eating in the evening. A recent trial tested this theory among a group of pre-diabetic men and the results were certainly impressive. All of the men's insulin sensitivity improved and their pancreatic beta-cells, which make insulin, became more responsive. Moreover, their blood pressure dropped, there were fewer damaging oxidants in their blood and they were less hungry.[18] However, the schedule was pretty demanding. Their eating window was a tiny six hours – between 8 a.m. and 2 p.m. – into which they had to squeeze three meals. Such a regime would wreak havoc with many people's schedules, and adjusting to it can take up to twelve days.

Fortunately, though, good results can still be achieved by following a less rigid timetable. Indeed, the flexibility of the IF diet is one of its principal advantages, and this also fits very neatly with the underlying principle of the Hybrid Diet: that switching between different metabolic states is crucial for the maintenance of good health.

Intermittent Fasting and Valter Longo's Fasting-Mimicking Diet

The most turbo-charged version of an IF diet is the 'fasting-mimicking diet'. This is designed to achieve all of the benefits of a traditional water fast, which turns on the body's repair processes and has been found to reduce biomarkers for ageing, diabetes, heart disease and cancer, with no adverse effects. It even has the potential to regrow parts of damaged organs and bring defunct insulin-producing beta-cells back to life.

The diet was developed by Professor Valter Longo, a biochemist and gerontologist at the University of Southern California. It was Longo's research that inspired Dr Michael Mosley to try a basic version of the 5:2 diet for his TV programme *Trust Me, I'm a Doctor*. The rest is diet-book history.

Longo emphasises the benefits of switching between metabolic states. He says his diet 'may help people to become more metabolically flexible. First, they switch to fat burning and start oxidising fatty acids for energy and then they switch back to more carbohydrates and glucose. So, you get accustomed to using both glucose and fatty acids as sources of energy.'

The fasting-mimicking diet is a five-day fast, during which participants eat between 700 and 1,000 calories per day, but with the same ratio of carbs, protein and fat (5–10, 20–25 and 70–80 per cent, respectively) as they would on a ketogenic diet. Longo has developed a kit with everything you need for those five days (see Resources), but the diet can also be done with any high fat foods, as long as they are eaten in the right proportions. (In our high fat phase, you would be in the right ballpark if you eliminated the snacks and had just two main meals per day, with neat C8 oil instead of the usual Hybrid Lattés. See Chapter 22.) The most intense way to use the diet is once a month, with the rest of the month spent recovering and refeeding (for example, in a slow carb phase).

'The changes it produces are much more pronounced than those caused by calorie restriction or an overnight fast,' says Longo. 'That's in part because it makes patients go into a fully ketogenic state *right away.*'

Many people who want to rejuvenate and repair their cells or lose a large amount of weight very quickly are now using Longo's diet. However, it is still experimental, and Longo himself says that it should only really be undertaken on medical advice because 'It is more sophisticated than people realize.'[19]

Several studies have thrown up some surprising results. One involving seventy-one people found the familiar and predictable changes in significant markers such as weight, blood pressure, blood glucose levels and total cholesterol.[20] However, 'What was remarkable', says Longo, 'was that those who were well – with low blood pressure, low triglycerides and low glucose – saw no change. That's very different to what happens with simple calorie restriction, which just keeps driving your markers down, whatever they are.'

Meanwhile, an animal trial found that repeated cycling

between the fasting-mimicking diet and a period of rest resulted in significant repair of beta-cells that had been badly damaged by insulin resistance.[21] If the diet has a similar effect in humans, it might prove valuable in reversing diabetes.

The Need for Exercise

Intermittent fasting or a ketogenic diet should always be combined with specific types of exercise, because, while cutting carbs and calories has positive health benefits (such as reducing high levels of glucose and insulin), it also puts your muscles under threat. This is because the rapid fall in carbs turns off the body's fat controller – mTOR – the enzyme that is responsible for muscle growth. In search of fresh supplies of glucose, the body turns to protein, which is found in the muscles, and breaks it down into its constituent amino acids. While this is happening, the best way to preserve muscle is through exercises that maintain and renew it. However, this is unlikely to be a concern if you go ketogenic for a week, but would be if you did it for a month.

Exercise makes it less likely that muscle will be transported to the liver for recycling into glucose because a resistance or strength workout – that is, exercises that are designed to build muscle – switches mTOR back on for a short period of time. Just eight minutes every other day is enough. The exercises can be done on gym machines or using rubber resistance bands; simple press-ups or exercises that make use of your body weight will also suffice.

Of course, when the body's mTOR is reactivated, you need sufficient protein in your diet to build muscle. Don't worry, though, we took this into consideration when formulating the Hybrid Diet (see Chapter 21). Also, remember that the fat controller is switched off by caffeine, so make sure you have your morning coffee at least thirty minutes before exercising. You'd be better off eating after exercise, and making sure there's protein in your meal.

If you do no strengthening/resistance exercises on a regular basis, you are likely to lose as much as 40 per cent of your muscle mass by the time you are eighty.[22] And you can ill-afford to do that, because muscle is needed for the production of several crucial chemicals that start to decline as you get older, including human growth hormone (hGh) – which may have anti-ageing benefits – testosterone and dehydroepiandrosterone (DHEA). Muscle is also more metabolically active than fat (that is, it burns far more calories), so if you lose muscle mass, you gain more weight, despite eating the same number of calories.

You also need to supplement resistance training with aerobic exercise – brisk walking, jogging, running, dancing or cycling (in short, anything that makes your heart beat faster and gets you sweating) – as this will strengthen your heart, burn calories and help you lose that dangerous belly fat. It also shortens the length of time it takes to initiate ketogenesis after starting a ketogenic diet because a good cardio workout stimulates the breakdown of glycogen to release the glucose that the muscles need. And you can enter ketosis only once all of the body's reserves of glycogen have been exhausted.

Finally, aerobic exercise raises metabolic rate for twenty-four hours, so you will benefit from increased fat burning for a whole day. The best time to do it is in the morning, before breakfast. During the high fat phase, if you fast for at least 14 hours (dinner at 6pm, breakfast at 10am) you're switching on autophagy. If you then do half an hour of aerobic exercise – enough to get you sweating – that will accelerate autophagy. Then have a breakfast that contains a source of protein, as that'll help you prevent muscle loss.

Interval Training

However, standard aerobic workouts don't do much for muscle building. What you need are short, sharp bursts of *flat out* activity. At first, this might involve alternating two minutes of low intensity walking with two minutes of brisk walking for a total of thirty minutes. Gradually, though, you might aim to build up to two minutes of walking and two minutes of jogging, then two minutes of jogging on the flat coupled with two minutes uphill, or two minutes of jogging and two minutes of hard running. Any or all of these can be done on a treadmill at the gym if it is more convenient. Cycling is another option.

As you get more experienced, you could sprint flat out for one minute, then switch to a gentle 'recovery' pace for three minutes, then go flat out again. However, you will need to do this at least half a dozen times per session to see any significant muscle-building effect.

Cardio and Strength Training – the Dynamic Duo

One of the simplest and most practical ways to achieve the best of both worlds is to stick to a weekly exercise routine that was developed by the former Gladiator Kate Staples (Zodiac). This comprises an eight-minute strengthening/resistance workout every other day and a thirty-minute cardio workout three times a week. A forty-five-minute brisk walk or cycle ride twice a week would also suffice. The eight-minute strengthening workout is composed of four exercises that vary in difficulty depending on whether you are a beginner, intermediate or advanced (for example, a full press-up is advanced), with each exercise done twice for one minute. All of the exercises can be done anywhere without any specialist equipment, although, as you advance, it might be worth investing in some hand weights, to take the place of water bottles. (See www.hybriddiet.co.uk/exercise.)

One word of caution: if you are combining low calories with a high fat ketogenic diet for up to a week, as in Longo's fasting mimicking diet (FMD – see page 140), any strength training you do should be light to moderate, not excessive, especially if you are not in the best of health or fitness. An eight-minute session every other day is more than enough. If you are unfit we'd recommend half this – four exercises each done for one minute. Two much strength training switches mTOR back on, and autophagy off. Don't overdo strength training when fasting. You are, after all, in a repair and renew phase, not a building phase.

Chapter 16

Breaking Sugar, Carb and Stimulant Addiction

Life is organised into cycles: day and night, awake and sleep, stimulated and relaxed, hungry and satisfied, growth and repair. Similarly, we have two energy systems – sugar/glucose and fat/ketones.

The 'digital revolution' has witnessed – and indeed precipitated – a plethora of changes, with the most profound relating to the pace of modern life. People all over the world – but especially in cities – are sleeping less, having less down time, feeling more anxious and stressed, and burning out at faster rates than ever before. All of these issues are reflected in sky-rocketing levels of absenteeism from work, depression and suicide.

The ubiquity of modern communication – in the form of emails, smartphones and digital media – leaves many of us feeling obliged to react instantly to ever-more demands that arrive at ever-increasing speed. The average person swipes their smartphone 2,600 times a day, including last thing at night and the moment they wake up in the morning. One US survey found that one in ten university students even check their smartphones *during* sex! Many people also suffer from nomophobia – a state of anxiety generated by the absence of a mobile phone signal.

All of this frenetic activity and anxiety place enormous demands on the body's energy supplies, and many people turn to caffeine, sugar and fast food just to keep going. In our 100% Health questionnaire – which has now been completed by almost 100,000 people – an ever-increasing number of respondents admit to:

- Feeling anxious, panicky, overwhelmed or stressed

- Inadequate sleep due to an inability to fall asleep or waking up too early

- Mood dips

- A sensation of running on empty

- Problems with concentration and an inability to stay calm and focused

- A 'need' for coffee, sugar, nicotine, alcohol, drugs (illegal or prescribed) and/or digital connection

- An overriding urge to buy or consume in order to feel good

- Feeling out of control and lost

If you experience any (or possibly all) of these issues, the chances are that your brain has been hijacked and you don't even know it. We are living in Space Age times with Stone Age minds, and companies selling everything from junk food to social media have learned how to exploit this evolutionary lag to boost their profits. In short, they know how to get us hooked on their products by manipulating the brain's antiquated 'reward system'. This is also part of the reason why prescriptions for antidepressants, sleeping pills and tranquillisers have gone through the roof. UK prescriptions for antidepressants alone have gone up eightfold in twenty years, from 8 million in 1998 to 65 million in 2017. A recent report on antidepressants found that over half of those taking these drugs suffered side effects, many serious, when they tried to stop but almost none were warned about this.[23]

The brain's reward system is based on the release of dopamine, which gives us a short burst of wellbeing and satisfaction when we get what we want. It's like slot-machine addiction: you continue to invest in the hope of hitting the jackpot. And clever marketing techniques keep us interested. Facebook, for example, uses prompts, swipe downs and red icons that we are encouraged to click in order to find out if we've 'won' and to get that lovely dopamine hit. Has a posting received a 'like'? Do I have more 'friends'? Has another person 'linked' to me on LinkedIn?

How your brain becomes addicted

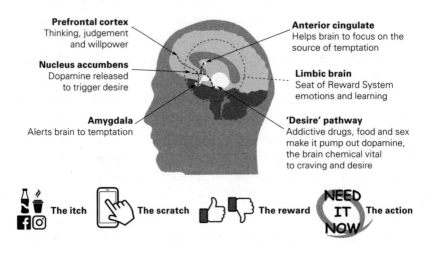

Prefrontal cortex
Thinking, judgement and willpower

Nucleus accumbens
Dopamine released to trigger desire

Amygdala
Alerts brain to temptation

Anterior cingulate
Helps brain to focus on the source of temptation

Limbic brain
Seat of Reward System emotions and learning

'Desire' pathway
Addictive drugs, food and sex make it pump out dopamine, the brain chemical vital to craving and desire

The itch   The scratch   The reward   The action

All of this means that your brain is being continually, insidiously and unwittingly lured into addiction, and not only by the social media giants. Gambling, gaming, food and pharmaceutical companies all entice us with similar techniques.

Hooked on Sugar

Sugar triggers the reward system to release dopamine, but overuse leads to reward deficiency. In this sense, it is similar to heroin or cocaine.[24] Dr Candace Pert, Research Professor in the Department of Physiology and Biophysics at Georgetown University Medical Center in Washington DC and the author of *The Molecules of Emotion*, was the first person to state this explicitly: 'I consider sugar to be a drug,' she wrote, 'a highly purified plant product that can become addictive. Relying on an artificial form of glucose – sugar – to give us a quick pick-me-up is analogous to, if not as dangerous as, shooting heroin.'[25] At the time, this comparison was greeted with cries of derision. Now, however, most people accept that sugar is indeed highly addictive.

In addition, Paul Kenny, whom we met in Chapter 13, found that rats' reward systems become ever more depressed as their weight increases.[26] Exactly the same thing happens with cocaine and heroin addiction: the body's dopamine receptors become insensitive. This is known as 'dopamine resistance', which is akin to insulin resistance. When Kenny fed rats 'cafeteria' food – high in both sugar and fat – they became compulsive eaters, searching for that feel-good effect but increasingly unable to find it.[27] Like all addictions, you crave more and more but experience less and less reward, until you have to keep guzzling just to not feel terrible. By that point, you're hooked.

Under normal circumstances, if you haven't eaten for a while, your blood sugar dips and the adrenal glands release appetite and 'hunter' hormones. These induce a highly stimulated mood, which our ancestors needed before setting off on a potentially dangerous hunt. Your whole body is motivated to do whatever is necessary to find food . . . and when you finally find it, those first few mouthfuls taste really good! As the saying goes, 'Hunger is the best sauce.' When you've eaten your fill, the body's appetite control mechanism kicks in. The adrenal hormones dissipate and you feel satisfied and relaxed. Time for a siesta, perhaps!

As we saw in Chapter 13, when Paul Kenny's rats were fed *either* a high fat diet *or* a high carb diet, their normal appetite controls eventually kicked in and they stopped eating.[28] However, when he fed them half fat and half (fast) carbs, they just kept going. He even tried to stop them by administering electric shocks: 'We then warned the rats as they were eating – by flashing a light – that they would receive a nasty foot shock. Rats eating the bland chow would quickly stop and scramble away, but time and again the obese rats continued to devour the rich food, ignoring the warning they had been trained to fear. Their hedonic desire overruled their basic sense of self-preservation.' As with alcoholics and drug addicts, the more the rats ate, the more they wanted.

This happens because overeaters become increasingly dopamine resistant over time: that is, their dopamine receptors start to shut down. In addition, Kenny has found that obese people, like drug addicts, have fewer dopamine D2 receptors (D2Rs) than people of a healthy weight,[29] and that some of them are born with this deficiency. In other words, you can be genetically predisposed to overeat.

Researchers at Brookhaven National Laboratory and the Oregon Research Institute discovered that obese people's reward systems respond weakly to all food, including junk food.[30] The muted pay-off they receive from eating then depresses mood. And how do they try to overcome this melancholia? By eating more and more of their favourite foods to gain that modest boost more often. It's a vicious cycle. The researchers concluded that obese people overeat to experience a fraction of the pleasure that lean individuals enjoy from much less food.

Nicole Avena of the University of Florida and others have found that particular fats or sugars, combinations of sugars and fats, and possibly salt are all highly addictive.[31] Meanwhile, a study by Professor David Ludwig of Boston Children's Hospital suggests that highly processed, quickly digested fast carbs can trigger cravings.[32] But no single ingredient stokes food addiction better than the high calorie combination of fat and sugar. As we pointed out in Chapter 13, this is not a natural combination; it is a product of the modern food industry. Sure, there are plenty of examples of concentrated sugar (such as honey) in nature, as well as concentrated fats and oils, but never equal proportions of the two in a single foodstuff. By contrast, the archetypal modern industrial food – the doughnut – is almost exactly half fat and half carbohydrate.

Given that our metabolism is designed to run on *either* glucose from carbs *or* ketones from fat, things start to go wrong if you supply – and especially if you oversupply – both simultaneously. According to Paul Kenny, 'modern high-calorie foods can overwhelm our biological feedback networks in a way that other foods cannot'.

Ketogenic and Slow Carbs Are the Best Ways to Beat Addiction

Whether you have become addicted to sugar, food, caffeine or perpetual digital stimulation, are unable to switch off without alcohol, have trouble sleeping, or have slipped into 'recreational' drug use, such as cocaine or a cocktail of uppers and downers, your brain's reward system has been hijacked and you will probably find it difficult to stick to *any* diet – be it a conventional calorie-counting approach, low GL or ketogenic.

But at least the main rule of the ketogenic diet is clear – no carbs! With some group support, you should be able to make it through the initial 'withdrawal' phase, during which your brain's dopamine resistance gradually subsides and normal appetite mechanisms start to re-emerge. An extreme version of this would be fasting, which should also be undertaken with support, if possible. It might be helpful to think of both fasting and the ketogenic diet as forms of rehab: the first few days are sure to be tough, but it'll get easier. The slow carb, low GL diet will also eventually reactivate the body's normal appetite mechanisms.

However, it should be remembered that addicted brains have been starved of essential nutrients for months or even years. Consequently, although your stocks of these biochemicals will gradually increase on either the ketogenic or the low GL diet, it may be beneficial to supplement them in order to speed up the recovery process.

Reclaim Your Brain

Dr Joan Mathews Larson, author of the best-seller *Seven Weeks to Sobriety*, once said, 'If you've scrambled your brain, sitting in a group and talking about it won't unscramble your brain.' Her nutrition-based recovery programme recommended a precise diet backed up with supplements of nutrients and amino acids. The results were second to none in the treatment of alcoholics, and the same principle applies to food, sugar, caffeine and even digital media addictions.

The neurotransmitter dopamine is made from the amino acid tyrosine. Serotonin, another neurotransmitter that plays a key role in the brain's reward system – at least when it is functioning correctly – is made from the amino acid tryptophan. N-acetyl cysteine and GABA are other amino acids that help to mitigate overstimulation. The mineral chromium improves insulin sensitivity and mood while lowering sugar cravings (see page 280).[33] Niacin (B$_3$), vitamin C, B vitamins, magnesium are all essential in the proper functioning of the reward system, too.

Three important experiments highlighted the importance of these nutrients in overcoming addiction. The first gave an amino acid supplement (NAC) or a placebo to fifteen hospitalised cocaine addicts, then measured the patients' desire for the drug. Those on the supplement reported much less desire, and showed much less interest in slides that showed cocaine and cocaine use.[34]

In the second study, researchers from the Department of Psychiatry at the University of Minnesota's School of Medicine gave pathological gamblers NAC supplements for eight weeks. More than half of the participants reported a significantly reduced urge to gamble. In the second half of the trial, the gamblers were given either NAC or a placebo. More than 80 per cent who received NAC reported even fewer urges to gamble, while more than 70 per cent who received the dummy pill resumed their previous gambling habits.[35]

In the third study, Professor Kenneth Blum from the University of Texas gave amino acid supplements to a group of outpatient carbohydrate bingers who had enrolled in a weight-control programme at the Bariatric Medical Clinic, Louisiana. Those who took the supplement for ninety days lost an average of 27lb and had a relapse rate of only 18 per cent. A control group in the weight-loss programme who were not given the supplement lost an average of 10lb but had a relapse rate of 82 per cent.[36]

Supplementing the right nutrients helps to reset the body's reward system and speeds up recovery from addiction by taking the edge off the cravings that can develop when you switch to a new diet that is devoid of sugar and fast carbs – be it ketogenic or low GL. It also helps to reduce cravings for caffeine and allows you to reclaim your natural sense of connection and contentment, clarity of mind and purpose, and ability to sleep like a baby and wake up fully charged and refreshed.

The key amino acids are tyrosine and tryptophan – the main constituents of dopamine and serotonin, respectively. When our overwrought reward system becomes depressed, we become dopamine depleted and adrenally exhausted. Tyrosine is also a building block or precursor of adrenalin (the fast-acting stress hormone), noradrenalin (which is associated with more positive states of stress) and the 'energy' hormone thyroxine. The level of another adrenal hormone – cortisol – increases in periods of prolonged stress, but in chronic stress, when we can no longer cope, it also becomes depressed. Meanwhile, the 'good' stress hormone – DHEA – and the 'happy' neurotransmitter – serotonin – are depleted. When this happens, you feel less natural joy and little sense of connection. As a result, serotonin depletion is viewed as a major cause of depression.

Of course, the pharmaceutical conglomerates are well aware of this. Consequently, most of the antidepressants they produce are serotonin reuptake inhibitors, noradrenalin reuptake inhibitors, or a combination of the two. Cocaine and Ritalin (methylphenidate) are both dopamine reuptake inhibitors, which means that they stop the body recycling this critical neurotransmitter. This gives a short-term boost but ultimately leaves the user more depleted, and hence more dependent on the drug. As a result, users can suffer serious side effects when they attempt to come off it. It's good for business, but often not so great for the person involved.

So, why not restore the brain's natural balance by supplementing natural amino acids? For the pharmaceutical industry, the answer is simple: money! You can't patent a naturally occurring chemical.

But does supplementing work? Consider an experiment conducted by Oxford University's Department of Psychiatry.[37] Fifteen women were given a diet devoid of tryptophan, the main constituent of serotonin. Within eight hours, ten of them started to feel depressed. However, when tryptophan was reintroduced to their diet, without their knowledge, their mood improved. This is how quickly what you eat affects how you feel.

At the time of writing, twenty-eight studies had explored the use of 5-HTP (another precursor of serotonin that is produced from tryptophan) in the treatment of depression. Most of these trials concluded that it works as well as or better than the leading commercial antidepressants, with minimal side effects.[38] This is important research, because antidepressants have been linked to both suicidal and homicidal tendencies.[39] For instance, a TV documentary in the well-respected *Panorama* series titled 'A Prescription for Murder' suggested that such medications may have induced pathological behaviour that culminated in dozens of mass shootings in the United States.[40] Such adverse reactions may be rare, but doesn't it make sense to explore the potential of a natural, safer, equally or more effective alternative?

Soldiers are already given the other key amino acid – tyrosine – to boost their dopamine and help them cope with combat stress. Meanwhile, many stimulant and alcohol addicts have extreme dopamine resistance, meaning that their receptors are malfunctioning, which is why their cravings are so strong. Indeed, we all increase our dopamine resistance through too much stimulation. That's why we 'need' ever more food, drink or social media likes and retweets to feel good . . . or at least normal.

However, this constant craving can be overcome in about a month with the right nutritional support, diet and lifestyle adjustments. You will find that you start to experience more control and less stress. You will restore a healthy balance between work and rest, waking and sleeping. Just as the Hybrid Diet places you in control of your metabolism and allows you to switch seamlessly between running on glucose and running on ketones, which gives your body a chance to repair and rejuvenate, it allows your brain to switch between states of healthy stimulation and rejuvenating connection and relaxation.

Anti-Addiction Actions

Whether you just want to break a stubborn sugar addiction or would like to go the whole hog and escape from the endless cycle of perpetual consumption, the following actions will help.

- For sugar addiction, supplement the mineral chromium, which comes in 200mcg tablets. Take one tablet one to three times a day with meals. Chromium can also boost mood, and if it has this effect on you, try taking three tablets a day. You have plenty of scope to experiment as the toxic level is 10,000mcg a day.

- For all addictions, or if you feel burned out, take an amino acid supplement that provides both 5-HTP (100mg) and tyrosine (1,000mg), both of which are best absorbed on an empty stomach (see Resources). Take once tablet before breakfast and another in the afternoon. For more serious stimulant addictions, NAC (1,000mg) may help.

- If you crave coffee and feel completely flat if you don't have a cup first thing in the morning, you are probably dopamine and/or adrenalin resistant or depleted. A supplement containing 5-HTP (100mg) and tyrosine (1,000mg) will help you get over caffeine withdrawal. Some supplements also contain the adaptogenic herbs ginseng, Siberian ginseng, reishi mushroom and rhodiola, all of which are helpful too. See Resources.

- Have a maximum of one coffee a day, first thing in the morning, never with carbs, but with a dollop of coconut butter or full fat cream, or have a Hybrid Latté (see page 305). If you drink tea or green tea, use the original teabag for your second and third cups.

- Avoid all caffeinated drinks after midday. Caffeine depresses melatonin for up to ten hours, which makes it harder to sleep.

- If you can't sleep, try supplementing 5-HTP (which is a precursor of melatonin as well as serotonin), magnesium and theanine (the relaxing amino acid in tea). Alternatively, supplement melatonin (3mg) itself. The latter is available over the counter in the United States or on prescription from your doctor in the UK and the rest of Europe.

- If you find it hard to fall asleep, listen to John Levine's CD *Silence of Peace* in bed. This switches the brain's activity from stimulating beta-waves to relaxing alpha-waves.

- Get outdoors every day and ideally exercise. Both sunlight and exercise boost serotonin, so go for a walk or a bike ride in nature. And turn your phone off!

- If you are prone to feeling stressed and anxious, consider taking up meditation, yoga, t'ai chi or any activity that allows you to switch off for at least twenty minutes every day. Don't end your day watching the news, thrillers or horror films. Do something relaxing like having a bath infused with lavender or read a book.

- Learn to recognise the signs of social media addiction, such as checking Facebook the minute you wake up and while lying in bed at night.

- Try not to obsess about making as many friends or getting as many likes as you can. Start questioning what you are doing on social media and how much of your activity on it is worthwhile. Try giving it up for a week and see how you feel. Look for ways to use it more constructively.

Chapter 17

Going Hybrid Makes Evolutionary Sense

Why did we become hybrid? Why did evolution decide that we needed to derive energy from *both* glucose *and* ketones? Some animals can't do this at all, but we are extremely good at it. In addition, as we have seen, human babies run on ketones from the moment they are born until several months after they finish breastfeeding. What benefits do they derive from meeting their energy requirements in this way?

All species survive because they thrive on a particular diet and develop a set of characteristics and skills that allow them to establish themselves in a specific environment. Clues to our ideal diet and environment can be found in the human brain. It's not just the brain's size but its complexity and highly developed frontal cortex that set us apart from other species. Infants make a staggering one million new neural connections every *second*,[41] and their brains burn through 75 per cent of the energy they use.

To fuel this furious growth, they need to top up their supplies of glucose from the moment they arrive in the world. They get this extra energy from ketones, which they make from breast milk and their own reserves of fat. By contrast, less intelligent mammals, such as bears, turn their stored fat into a form of glucose (glycerol) during hibernation. Their smaller brains have lower energy demands, so they don't need to bother with ketones. Meanwhile, the larger brains of dolphins and seals are similar to our own. Indeed, they prefer to run on ketones, rather than glucose, if the former are available.

We didn't survive on the savannah because we started to stand upright and throw spears. Our muscles are, frankly, puny compared to those of other animals. And even lions, whose bulging muscles, strength and speed are far superior to ours, don't have a particularly good strike rate during hunts. Therefore, we needed to increase our chances of securing a meal through intelligence, not muscle power. Key to this had to be our ability to convert omega-3 into DHA, one of the main building blocks of all mammalian brains.

For that we needed a much richer source of omega-3 – along with selenium and iodine – if our brains were ever to grow into the super-computers that they are today. That meant we had to make our way to the water's edge.

Homo Aquaticus

Genetically, we are quite close cousins of chimpanzees. Our family trees diverged a mere seven million years ago, and we share 98.5 per cent of the same genes. Yet, in other respects, we are utterly different. So, how did this happen? The answer is that we spent a lot of time in – or next to – the water, while chimpanzees did not.

We all have a layer of subcutaneous fat: human babies, unlike all other land mammals, are born with lots of it. In addition, we have a larger brain to body weight ratio and a much higher concentration of omega-3 fatty acids (such as DHA) in our brains than any other mammal as well as an ability to convert fat into ketones rapidly. Moreover, as we saw earlier, we continue to use ketones for brain fuel long after weaning. We also have a remarkable 'swimming reflex'. Babies just a few months' old know how to 'dive' into the water, hold their breath while they are below the surface, then start breathing again when they pop back up. While underwater, they stay calm, open their eyes and even know how to roll over onto their backs without the water going up their noses. And we are all born with a coating of vernix – a waxy, waterproof layer. No other land mammals have this trait, shared with seals.

All of this, coupled with the fact that we walk upright, on two legs, gave us a unique evolutionary advantage to thrive in a specific environment. 'The niche that ultimately made us human was coastal areas, rivers and wetlands – the water's edge,' says Professor Michael Crawford, Director of the Institute of Brain Chemistry and Human Nutrition and a champion of the '*Homo aquaticus*' theory, which is supported by an ever-increasing body of evidence. The argument is that our ancestors left the jungles and savannahs of central Africa and made their way to the water's edge, most likely the stretch of coastline that now runs from Eritrea in the north-east of the continent to South Africa. This coast was – and still is – fringed by reefs that hold an abundance of seafood.

Crawford suggests that our ancestors simply waded into the shallow water and helped themselves to the mussels, oysters, crustaceans and fish, which provided the copious supplies of omega-3s and other critical nutrients that allowed our brains to grow to an unprecedented size. Neither a vegetarian nor a meat-based diet provides these nutrients in anything like the same quantities, so it is highly unlikely that the human brain would have developed as it did if our ancestors had not made that decisive move to the coast. In addition, their diet would have been much lower in carbs and higher in fat and protein than those of earlier generations, which would have had the effect of increasing their reliance on ketones.

The migration to the coast occurred about two million years ago, according to the fossil record. Thereafter, there was a steady growth in brain size from 450g to 1,490g, which *Homo sapiens* achieved about 100,000 years ago. Meanwhile, these early humans also evolved a much more upright posture than their savannah-dwelling ancestors (and indeed the chimps that remained there). The evolutionary advantages of this upright stance are obvious, given where they were living and what they were eating: it allowed them to wade further into the coastal lagoons for the richest pickings.

About 1.8 million years ago, after a few hundred thousand years of rapid mental and physical development on the East African coast, *Homo erectus* started to explore further afield. They reached the southern Mediterranean, the Middle East, India and East Asia. By then, the human brain had already doubled in size to 940g. Later, those who remained in – or possibly returned to – Africa ultimately evolved into *Homo sapiens*. Then, like their ancestors before them, they started to spread around the world, too. Recent archaeological discoveries in China, Israel and Morocco suggest that our species reached these places around 180,000 years ago.[42]

The most ancient rock art – which has been dated to around 80,000 BCE – is in sub-Saharan Africa, which had a vast network of lakes, rivers and wetlands at the time. One particularly significant cave painting from this period shows a group of early humans swimming. Then weather patterns changed, the monsoon moved further south, and the whole area dried up. By 10,000 years ago, only the Nile was left. Further north, the Tigris and Euphrates (in modern-day Iraq) were similarly isolated water sources. It was along the banks of these rivers that human civilisation and culture started to flourish, and even today the vast majority of the world's major cities are on the water's edge.

Having identified our close connection with coasts and rivers throughout our evolutionary history, Michael Crawford laments the decline in omega-3 in our diet. Indeed, as early as 1972, he argued that we will become a race of morons if we continue to eat the modern Western diet. He warned of an ever-increasing incidence of mental illness, lower IQs and more children with ADHD, autism and other serious disorders. So, has this dire prediction come true? Well, mental illness is now the number-one global health issue and one recent study found that average IQ has fallen by seven points in a single generation.[43]

Babies Run on Ketones

Clearly, then, our ancestors' adaptation to a diet that included marine fats and extra protein – and their reduced reliance on carbs – was the key development that enabled our brains to grow much larger than those of other primates. An integral part of this process was that we honed our ability to run on ketones, because we needed to ensure that our expanding brains never ran out of fuel.

According to Professor Stephen Cunnane from the University of Sherbrook in Quebec, 'Ketones are the back-up fuel to glucose in the human adult, but in the neonate [infant] they are the predominant brain fuel.' While other large-brained animals have some capacity to convert fat into ketones, we are far better at it, and our babies – more than the offspring of any other land mammals – actually depend on them.

Campfires on the Beach

However, it wasn't just the fats and proteins in seafood that shaped our development. Another significant milestone was the discovery of fire about 1.8 million years ago. Thereafter, and especially after around 500,000 BCE, cooking had a huge impact on our ancestors' diet and evolution. It made previously hard to digest root vegetables and beans more edible and therefore valuable new sources of energy because of the low GL carbs they contain.

This coincided with a further and steady increase in brain size, along with a parallel increase in aerobic capacity, a shortening of the gut and a reduction in tooth size. A plausible explanation for all of these physiological changes is that cooking meant our ancestors needed to spend less time chewing food in the mouth as well as digesting and absorbing nutrients in the gut. Uncooked vegetables, meat and fish all demand a lot of chewing.

Our genes support this theory. About a million years ago, multiple variations in carbohydrate-digesting amylase enzymes – which turn cooked starch into glucose – started to appear. This meant that more fuel was available for both the body and the brain. 'Consumption of increased amounts of starch may have provided a substantial evolutionary advantage to Mid-to-Late Pleistocene omnivorous hominins,' according to Karen Hardy and Jenny Brand-Miller from the University of Sydney.[44] Cooked starch – a rich source of preformed glucose – greatly increased energy availability to human tissues with high glucose demands, including the brain, red blood cells and developing foetuses.

By 20,000 BCE, the hunter-gatherer *Homo sapiens'* diet consisted chiefly of lean meat, fish and shellfish, eggs, vegetables and fruit. Some wild lentils, grasses, grains and peas may have been eaten too, but these foodstuffs didn't take off in a major way until the Agricultural Revolution, more than 10,000 years later. There was no consumption of dairy products, and of course no processed food.

There are still some so-called hunter-gatherers in the world, although most of these tribes are actually pastoralists who rear cattle, which is a relatively recent development. The Tsimane tribe in the Peruvian Amazon are among the very few who follow a more prehistoric lifestyle. They get 72 per cent of their calories from the unrefined, high fibre (and hence low GL) carbohydrates in rice, plantain, manioc, corn, nuts and fruits. Protein comprises 14 per cent of their diet, mainly from lean animal meat and fish, such as wild pigs, piranha, catfish and the occasional monkey. Their fat intake is low – just 14 per cent – far less than the average Western diet. They have the lowest risk of heart disease in the world: even those over the age of seventy-five have virtually no cardiovascular problems or hardening of the arteries. The Hadza in Tanzania have a very similar diet and they are just as healthy. However, before you decide to follow suit, bear in mind that both of these tribes burn a lot of calories through exercise. The average Tsimane man hunts for around six to seven hours each day, while the average woman gathers and prepares food for four to five hours. All of this is hard physical activity.

There is a rather meat-centric myth about our ancestors, but in reality hunting for animals was always a rather hit-and-miss affair. Consequently, the (usually male) hunter needed support from a (usually female) forager. It was only much later in our evolutionary history, when we started to domesticate animals, that meat became a widespread 'staple' of the human diet.

The diets of the Masai and Samburu tribes in East Africa have remained largely unchanged since that time. During the dry season, they live almost exclusively on beef, blood and a little milk as they roam the savannah in search of water for their cattle, which forces their bodies to burn ketones for energy. When the rains return, they become less nomadic, set up camp, and switch to a more varied, mostly plant-based diet, which includes more daily carbs. Although this is healthier than the modern Western diet, it is far from optimal, and certainly a significant departure from the coastal diet of our prehistoric ancestors, which gave us so many evolutionary advantages. In short, while our bodies can live on meat, they are *designed* to thrive on fish and shellfish.

The Agricultural Revolution

Glaciers started to recede around 20,000 years ago, which allowed 'plant species previously confined to sheltered habitats ... to spread well beyond their regions of origin', according to Ivan Crowe in his book *The Quest for Food*.[45] These were favourable conditions for the wild grains that our ancestors were already eating. Wheat, barley and lentils all grew well along the shores of the Sea of Galilee, where archaeologists have found evidence of early pestles and mortars, used for grinding.

Many people think that humans 'chose' to start farming around 12,000 years ago. However, it may have had more to do with climate change: the very cold conditions of the last Ice Age were followed by drought, which drove tribes into Mesopotamia and the Nile Basin. These migrants carried grains from their places of origin and planted them in the fertile soil in order to survive.

The grains that grew most successfully were 'sticky' – high in gluten – and had a protective covering called chaff, which had to be removed as part of the harvesting and cleaning processes. Prime examples are wheat, rye and barley, which became mainstays of the Mesopotamian diet by about 9,000 BCE. Meanwhile, less robust – relatively low gluten – cereals were discarded.

The widespread cultivation of grain, and especially wheat, facilitated the formation of villages and then towns as tribes abandoned their traditional nomadic lifestyles and settled down. The invention of ploughing led to higher yields. Grain stores provided more security during winters and droughts. Domesticated animals began to appear around 6,000 BCE, starting with goats. As a result, consumption of meat and especially dairy products increased enormously. Rapid population growth ensued. Peasant farmers survived better than hunter-gatherers and claimed ever more of the most fertile land for themselves. The pace of civilisation accelerated as the food supply became increasingly stable.

The New Foods

The principal products of the Agricultural Revolution – wheat and milk – now account for a third of the calories in a typical Western diet.

As mentioned above, the Mesopotamians domesticated goats, whose milk and especially cheese are very high in butyric acid, a healthy pre-ketone that is good for the gut. Industrially produced cow's milk is rather different. Genetically, there are two different kinds of cow's milk – A1 and A2. Today, we mainly drink A1, which is produced by cows with the highest milk yields. Nile Basin cows, yaks and Jersey cows all produce smaller amounts of A2. Yet, A1 generates digestive discomfort in a much larger proportion of the population as well as inflammation in both lactose tolerant and intolerant individuals. In other words, we seem to be less well adapted to drink A1 milk.[46]

Meanwhile, the earliest wheats – khorasan (also known as Kamut bulgur), emmer and durum – are genetically much simpler than modern wheat. They are known as tetraploid grains because they have just four sets of chromosomes, whereas modern wheat and spelt are hexaploid, having six sets. More than twenty studies have found that modern wheat promotes inflammation whereas Kamut khorasan does not.[47] For example, in a recent trial involving participants with non-alcoholic fatty liver disease – which is often found in diabetics – those eating Kamut khorasan not only improved their liver function but also halved their level of inflammation.[48] Similarly, eating modern wheat tends to exacerbate the symptoms of IBS,[49] whereas most sufferers are able to tolerate Kamut khorasan, even though it contains gluten.[50]

An estimated one in thirty people with digestive problems have coeliac disease – a severe intolerance to gluten – whereas approximately one in five are gluten-sensitive but not coeliacs. It is not known whether the prevalence of these ailments is due to the differences between modern and ancient wheats, the high proportion of gluten in the Western diet, or a combination of the two. However, natural selection probably meant that those people who could not tolerate wheat of any kind died out in the Middle East between 10,000 and 2,000 years ago, leaving behind a population who could eat it quite happily. By contrast, wheat was unknown in the Northern European diet in that period, so no such natural selection took place. This may explain why gluten intolerance is such a problem in Northern Europe and other Western countries – but not in the Middle East – today.

Similarly, nomadic herdsmen in Africa suffer little of the lactose intolerance that blights the lives of so many Westerners. Their ancestors were among the first humans to start herding cattle, so those who were able to digest milk efficiently enjoyed a huge evolutionary advantage over the rest. Consequently, over time, these tribes became characterised by their tolerance for dairy products. Cattle herders in Europe and the Middle East evolved in a similar way. By contrast, societies with no ancient tradition of cattle rearing – such as the Chinese, Thai, Pima Indians of the American Southwest and the Bantu of West Africa – all have very high rates of lactose intolerance.

The Loss of Food Diversity

The earliest complex civilisations – those of the Sumerians and the Egyptians – emerged around 6,000 and 5,000 years ago, respectively. Both of them were based on the cultivation of grains, with the Sumerians growing barley, emmer and Kamut khorasan as well as beans, peas and lentils. Since then, cereals have been closely associated with virtually every highly developed civilisation around the world, including the Greeks, Romans and Babylonians. However, it is often forgotten that these societies also consumed large amounts of fish and shellfish, which gave them plenty of omega-3s as well as other marine food-rich vitamins and minerals. We could do the same, but we have increasingly neglected these foods in favour of high yield grains, meat and dairy products.

Humans can eat approximately 195,000 different plants quite safely, yet we choose to consume fewer than 300 species. Even more startlingly, a mere seventeen plant species now provide 90 per cent of our food, with eight cereal grains – wheat, maize, rice, barley, sorghum, oats, rye and millet – accounting for a massive 56 per cent of our total calorific intake, as well as half of all the protein that is consumed on earth. Moreover, just three crops – wheat, maize and rice – comprise at least three-quarters of the world's total grain production. These were generally eaten as whole grains until industrial refining processes – such as the milling of white flour – became widespread in the late nineteenth century. Today, for large chunks of humanity, grains stand between them and starvation.

Paleo, Vegan and Ketogenic Diets

The so-called 'paleo' diet is full of whole foods – vegetables, fruit, nuts, seeds, eggs, fish and 'healthy' lean meat. It shuns grains, beans and dairy products on the basis that these are all recent interlopers in humankind's evolutionary history. (Although some paleo people make an exception for peas, which are members of the bean family, because there is evidence that our close cousins, the Neanderthals, ate them at least 46,000 years ago.) It is also quite meat oriented, as are most ketogenic diets, although it has no particular problem with fish. The standard Atkins diet is especially high in meat and dairy products.

Vegans avoid all meat, eggs, fish and dairy products. The decision to adopt such a radical diet is entirely understandable ethically, given the terrible ways in which animals are reared, treated and slaughtered; environmentally, as it is more economical to grow a field of beans than feed a herd of cows; and politically, as it cocks a snook at the unscrupulous food manufacturers that are more interested in boosting their profits than safeguarding their customers' health. As Michael Crawford says, 'If you eat obese animals, you're going to get obese. In today's animals, there are six times more calories from fat than protein. The balance of nutrients is all wrong. Chicken are sold without the skin – which is rich in fat, flavour and nutrients – because more money can be made elsewhere, selling the skin, which is processed to add flavour to manufactured foods.' Many vegans and vegetarians adopt their diets because they are appalled by these gross perversions of factory meat farming and the dairy industry.

Unfortunately, though, for all their merits, there are some significant problems with vegan diets, especially for those who switch without any knowledge of nutrition. For instance, vegans find it particularly difficult to get enough vitamin B_{12} (which is non-existent in the vegetable kingdom), DHA (the key omega-3 fat, which is essential for brain development), vitamin D (which is found in high concentrations in fish) and selenium (which is also rich in seafood). The highly respected Avon Longitudinal Study found that the children of vegans – and others who eat little seafood – have below average cognition and social development,[51] while their mothers suffer from more anxiety during pregnancy.[52] The human body simply cannot convert flax seeds into sufficient quantities of DHA to facilitate optimal foetal brain development. Therefore, in our opinion, it is essential for vegans to supplement either omega-3 fish oils or DHA derived from seaweed throughout pregnancy and breastfeeding. Similarly, eggs are among the best sources of phospholipids, which are also vital to brain development.

Fans of paleo diets often highlight the advantages of eating grass-fed cattle rather than intensively reared, carb-fed cows. However, while beef from animals fed on high carb corn is certainly more marbled, fattier and therefore less healthy than the grass-fed alternative, even the latter is not truly paleo, if the intention is to replicate the diets of our hunter-gatherer forebears. It was much later in our evolutionary journey that a few tribes had the idea of keeping hoofed animals in a pen and forcing them to eat grass. In addition to being genetically very different from all modern cows – organically reared and grass-fed or otherwise – these animals were forest-dwellers and their natural diet consisted of hedges and bushes. A prehistoric hunter-gatherer might spear or snare one of these lean, wild beasts every once in a while, but his daily diet would consist primarily of fish, shellfish and plants.

Many ketogenic advocates insist that, while protein and fat are essential food groups, carbohydrates are not. However, there is a flaw in this argument because it is impossible to consume sufficient quantities of many nutrients – including antioxidants and polyphenols – if you swear off all carbs for good. Indeed, it is much more accurate to say that dairy products are not an essential food group. Moreover, they had no place in 99 per cent of our evolutionary history, so it is hardly surprising that half of the world's population are lactose intolerant. Yet, countless ketogenic enthusiasts make dairy an integral part of their diet.

Whether you are a fan of ketogenic, paleo, low carb or low GL, the chances are that you have a burning desire to eat unadulterated wholefoods, rather than junk food or the meat of intensively reared animals. In addition, though, many studies have found that eating *any* red meat – irrespective of how the animal was reared – increases the risk of developing various cancers, diabetes and heart disease. Crucially, there is no corresponding risk from eating fish. Indeed, in general, the more fish and vegetables you eat, the lower your risk of contracting any of these illnesses. So, it might be time to bypass the butcher's and make your way to the fishmonger's instead.

Why Our Dual Fuel System Gave Us an Evolutionary Advantage

Throughout the course of human evolution, we have benefited from our ability to run on two fuels – glucose and ketones – for the following reasons:

- The metabolism of ketones has been critical for human infants' brain development.

- Our ancestors were able to survive in different times and places, despite the varying availability of plant and animal-based food.

- Our diverse diet gave us access to a wide variety of nutrients that were not available to other animals, which facilitated the unprecedented growth of the human brain. However, many of these nutrients do not feature in modern diets, so were are in danger of *devolving*, rather than evolving, if we continue down the same path. Indeed, this may happen much faster than most evolutionary processes. One recent study found that diabetics' genes are altered by the condition, so they may pass on susceptibility to the disease to the next generation.[53]

- We have not evolved to survive exclusively on plant-based food, which is why vegans should supplement key nutrients such as B_{12} and DHA. Fish and shellfish have long been important sources of brain-friendly nutrients and indeed may have been *the* key food group that made us human.

- We did not rely on a very narrow diet, such as one that was heavily reliant on grains and dairy products. Consequently, it is not a good idea to limit our options in this way today.

- Our ancestors ate a little unprocessed, lean meat but got most of their protein from seafood, which is packed with omega-3s that aid brain development. Today, many people eat too much (and much less healthy) meat, while consumption of fish and shellfish has fallen dramatically. We need to reverse this.

Therefore, from an evolutionary perspective, the hybrid approach – which derives energy from both low GL carbs and fat while conserving protein for essential growth and repair – makes perfect sense. In addition, there may be health advantages from replicating the vast majority of our evolutionary history by fasting and/or initiating ketogenesis from time to time.

Variety – in terms of eating a wide range of foods and switching between ketones and glucose for fuel – may indeed be the spice of a healthier life.

Chapter 18

Switching: Why, When and How?

In the Western world, most of us have never suffered the horrors of starvation. And we have spent almost all of our well-fed lives running on carbs and burning glucose, rather than ketones. However, as we have seen, our bodies derive significant health benefits from the cellular rejuvenation that occurs during autophagy (see Chapter 14) as well as from total and intermittent fasting (Chapter 15). Consequently, it makes sense to switch occasionally from the slow carb diet – which we consider the default part of the Hybrid Diet – to a high fat, low carbs diet, because this will give your carb engine a crucial break.

Of course, there is an argument for making the ketogenic approach your default diet, but as yet there is no evidence that it is better for either weight control or disease prevention than the slow carb, low GL diet. Moreover, we are concerned that less healthy versions – which include too much meat, dairy and protein – might have harmful effects, for example in relation to colorectal cancer. It is also quite restrictive. As Professor David Ludwig from Harvard Medical School says:

> For people with type 2 diabetes or related metabolic problems, very low carbohydrate diets, including the ketogenic diet, may offer an excellent long-term option. In some cases, a very low carbohydrate diet can reverse diabetes rapidly, without severe calorie deprivation. Much more research is needed into this area. But, despite their potentially dramatic effects, very low carbohydrate diets can be difficult to maintain over the long term. Replacing added sugars and refined starchy foods with unprocessed carbohydrate, healthful fats and proteins may provide many of the benefits of a very low carbohydrate diet, without having to eliminate an entire class of nutritious [and delicious] foods.

In any event, in general, our view is that it is advisable to switch from low GL to ketogenic from time to time in order to trigger autophagy, but not to turn off the mTOR network – and therefore cellular growth (see Chapter 13) – for too long or too often. However, exceptions may be made for specific diseases, be it epilepsy or brain cancer, where there are compelling reasons to remain ketogenic over the long term.

Also, if you want to kickstart either weight loss or diabetes recovery, it's certainly an option to remain in the high fat phase until you get your blood sugar under control. Carb addicted people often find it easier to abstain completely, rather than try to limit their carb intake. Although, that said, we have found that addiction to carbs dissipates naturally on the low GL diet, too (see Chapter 16).

A key goal in switching between ketogenic and slow carbs is to improve metabolic flexibility, which entails moving seamlessly from burning ketones to burning glucose, and maintaining a balanced blood glucose level when eating carbs. Much of this happens because you regain insulin sensitivity, but many other biochemical pathways are also boosted by shifting from high fat to low GL and back again.

As with your muscles and joints when you join a yoga class, these pathways may feel stiff and achy at first because you haven't used them for a while. That's why it takes most people up to a week to initiate ketogenesis in the high fat phase and another week to 'stabilise' their bodies in a state of ketosis. During this process, your glucose level might drop from 5mmol/l to less than 3mmol/l, which is an indication that you are fully 'fat adapted'. This is why we recommend following the ketogenic diet for at least two weeks the first time you try it. Thereafter, when you return to the high fat phase after some time back on the default low GL diet, you will adapt much more rapidly (perhaps in as little as two to three days) and will reap the full benefits within a week.

An even 'faster' way in is to fast for a day or two, or simply eat no carbs at all for twenty-four hours. For example, eat dinner at 6 p.m., have a coffee with a dollop of coconut butter at 8 a.m. the next morning, then a no-carb 'keto' shake or Hybrid Latté (see page 305) at 10 a.m., a no-carb lunch (such as salmon and kale or spinach sautéed in ghee or coconut butter, perhaps with pesto or tahini) at 2 p.m., a spoonful of C8 MCT oil mid-afternoon (see page 189), then dinner at 6 p.m. from one of our recipes. In this example, you effectively eat nothing for sixteen hours, and effectively eat no carbs for the full twenty-four hours.

Another way to speed up your entry into ketosis is to go for a run or a long walk the day before you intend to begin the high fat phase, because this will force your body to break down glycogen. This is what long-distance runners do during a marathon.

After two weeks in the high fat phase, it is really easy – and enjoyable – to switch back to the slow carb phase, because you will be able to eat many delicious foods that you have been avoiding for a fortnight.

If you want to accelerate weight loss – and are not feeling too hungry – you might want to consider skipping a snack or a meal, as this will usher your body into the modified fasting realm, or exercising more. However, bear in mind that a healthy mid-afternoon snack may be particularly important if you have done a lot of exercise earlier in the day, as it will help you resist temptation before your evening meal.

Thirty minutes of cardio exercise (which raises your heartbeat) every other day, combined with resistance exercise (which tones muscles) every other day, aids healthy weight loss. The cardio exercise raises your metabolic rate for up to twenty-four hours, meaning you burn more fuel even when resting, while the resistance exercise instructs your body to build muscle, thus preserving muscle mass.

The Dual Fuel Timetable

After your initial two weeks on the ketogenic diet, we recommend alternating three weeks of slow carbs with one week of high fat. This is the standard '3G:1K' routine of the Hybrid Diet. It means you will spend nine months a year running on glucose, and three months a year running of ketones. Our prehistoric ancestors may have done just that – eating carbs every spring, summer and autumn, and living primarily on fat (including their own subcutaneous reserves) in the winter months when fewer carbs were available.

Of course, if you lapse, perhaps over the festive season, you can always throw in an additional high fat phase to repair the damage.

While you will lose weight (by releasing body fat) in both phases, you will lose an additional 2–3kg (4–6lb) due to water loss during the high fat phase. This will return when you switch back to the slow carb phase, but don't worry, you're not gaining fat, just the water in your new reserves of glycogen. After this brief increase, your weight will resume its downward trajectory as you continue to convert fat into energy.

By experimenting and becoming increasingly proficient in both phases, you will learn what works best for you. We are all different. Some people find the high fat phase too restrictive. For instance, it is certainly harder to do if you are vegetarian (and virtually impossible if you are vegan). On the other hand, meat-lovers prefer it to the low GL phase. Either way, though, you will gain metabolic flexibility, reduce your risk of contracting a chronic disease and lose weight.

A simple experiment on Channel 4's *How to Lose Weight Well* illustrated this. Two overweight guys – Callum and Jake – tried a low GL diet and the ketogenic 'Banting' diet, respectively. Callum had to avoid anything with sugar in it: simply, if it said 'sugar' on the label, he was not allowed to eat or drink it. This was close to our slow carb phase, even though Callum learned nothing about his food choices' glycemic load. He lost just under 3 stones 12lb in four months. Meanwhile, Jake lost 4 stones 4lb on his low carb, high fat diet, which approximated our ketogenic phase. (He also enjoyed it, because he liked eating meat.) Therefore, the difference between the two approaches was marginal, especially when you factor in the 4–6lb rebound weight gain when the body's glycogen stores are replenished following a ketogenic diet.

Why Dual Fuel Works Best

The ketogenic diet puts into practice many recent discoveries relating to how our metabolic engine room actually works. But it makes sense to combine it with occasional fasting and eating slow carbs because this gives you the best of both worlds – glucose for growth and ketones for repair. Moreover, you will continue to burn fat throughout. This is the key to the Hybrid Diet's success.

In summary,

- Switching between a ketogenic state, induced by a high fat diet and/or fasting, and a slow carb phase, when the focus is on low GL foods, optimises the balance between growth and repair because it puts the body in full control over insulin, mTOR and autophagy.

- You must maintain the high fat diet for at least two weeks the first time you try it. Thereafter, one week per month is a good benchmark, with the rest of the time spent in the slow carb phase. However, we are all different and you will soon work out what suits you best.

- You can reduce the length of time it takes to initiate ketogenesis with a long session of aerobic exercise the day before you plan to begin the high fat phase; fasting for sixteen hours; or eating no carbs for twenty-four hours.

- You can incorporate intermittent fasting into either or both phases by skipping snacks or even a meal once, twice or three times a week in order to accelerate weight loss. (See Patrick's book *Burn Fat Fast* for more details.[54])

- Exercise is important, especially resistance/strength training during the high fat phase, to preserve and build muscle. Ideally, you should have a cardio workout every other day and a strength workout every other day, or combine the two with interval training.

Part 4

The Hybrid Diet

In this part, we will show you how to put the Hybrid Diet principles into practice. You will learn about the good fats, the slow carbs, what to eat in the high fat and low GL phases, how to get your protein intake right, the importance of support nutrients to accelerate your weight loss and health gains, how to measure what's happening in order to establish what works best for you and even how to 'biohack' your system.

Chapter 19

Good Fats

As a food group, fat has been more maligned and misunderstood than any other. The demonisation of saturated fat and cholesterol – and especially the incorrect accusation that they are the main drivers of heart disease – has resulted in almost universal fat phobia that is hard to shake.

You will increase your intake of a variety of good fats in both the low GL and ketogenic phases of the Hybrid Diet. We call these 'good' either because they are essential for your health or because they are valuable sources of energy. However, you will eat different amounts in the two phases.

When you are on the ketogenic diet, fat will be your primary fuel, so you will need to choose the foods that are best for that (see page 227). Some fats are easier to burn, while others are easier to store. This is determined by two characteristics of the food in question: the length of its fat molecules – that is, short, medium or long chain – with short being the easiest to burn; and the number of 'unsaturated' gaps in the molecules. The illustration overlead demonstrates this.

Understanding the dynamics of fats

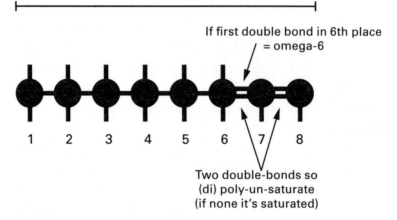

8 carbons long so C8 - medium chain triglyceride (MCT)

If first double bond in 6th place = omega-6

1 2 3 4 5 6 7 8

Two double-bonds so (di) poly-un-saturate (if none it's saturated)

Fats can be:

- Saturated, which are solid at room temperature (e.g. butter, lard, coconut oil and palm nut oil).

- Mono-unsaturated – one degree of unsaturation (oleic acid – e.g. olive oil).

- Di-unsaturated– two degrees of unsaturation (linoleic acid – e.g. sunflower oil).

- Tri-unsaturated– three degrees of unsaturation (linolenic acid – e.g. flax oil).

- 'Poly-unsaturated' is an umbrella term for any fat with more than one degree of unsaturation.

Poly-unsaturated fats can either be omega-3 or omega-6. The most unsaturated fats are the most biologically active, but they also contain more molecular gaps where oxidisation or hydrogenation can take place. The latter turns the fat into a 'trans fat', which looks like the real thing but doesn't work biologically. At one time, fats were deliberately hydrogenated to make them solid at room temperature. These manmade products were then used as replacements for the vilified (but entirely natural) saturated fats in cooking and the food industry. This was the basis of margarine, which could be considered a form of omega-6, since it is derived from sunflower oil. However, the fat stops working biologically after hydrogenation, so it is actually fake omega-6. Therefore, avoid it.

By far the most anti-inflammatory fats are undamaged omega-3s, followed by undamaged omega-6s. (However, note that some omega-6s, such as arachidonic acid, which is found in dairy products and meat, are inflammatory. People with insulin resistance, such as diabetics, find it difficult to turn omega-6 into its anti-inflammatory form.) The basic omega-3s are found in flax seeds, chia seeds, walnuts and, to some extent, pumpkin seeds and pecans, as well as hemp, although they are too hard to eat unless ground. Chia seeds have the highest concentration and they are tasty as well as high in soluble fibre and antioxidants, so they are the best all-rounders. However, all of these seeds and nuts, as well as their oils, are good to eat and low in carbs. An excellent source of omega-6 is tahini (sesame seed paste) – a dairy-free alternative to butter.

The most potent of all the omega-3s are DHA and EPA. As we saw in Part 3, the former is a key component in brain growth and development, while the latter has excellent anti-inflammatory properties, which means it is good for the cardiovascular system, joints, skin and gut. You get both from eating oily fish or fish that swim in cold water and eat other fish, or by supplementing their oil. (Cod liver oil is an exception. Cod is a white, non-carnivorous fish, but its liver oil is still a good source of omega-3.) Therefore, eating more mackerel, kippers, herrings, salmon, trout, sardines and fresh tuna – maybe in place of red meat, especially in the ketogenic phase – is a great way to boost your omega-3 while maintaining your intake of high-quality protein. Fortunately, vegetarians can derive sufficient amounts of EPA and DHA from seaweed or algae (seaweed is a type of algae that clings to the ocean floor, while other algaes float). Supplements are available.

Olive Oil and Oleic Acid

Oleic acid is not an essential fat, but it will do you no harm. Olive oil is the richest source and it has many proven health benefits, although these are not related to oleic acid. Rather, they are due to its significant quantities of omega-6, phytonutrients, which act as antioxidants, polyphenols and other anti-inflammatory agents. However, quality is crucial, and quite a lot of cheap, commercial brands are not even 100 per cent olive oil. Indeed, one study found that 70 per cent of olive oils are 'fake'.[1] Good-quality olive oil will go solid in the fridge far faster than these fake oils.

The really good stuff is so high in anti-inflammatory polyphenols that it protects blood lipids from oxidative stress, which helps to keep 'bad' LDL cholesterol low. We don't advocate the use of very high-quality olive oil during cooking, partly because it is so expensive. Therefore, add it to cooked foods, or use in salad dressings. Nevertheless, for cooking, use virgin cold-pressed olive oil, rather than one of the cheap brands.

Olive oil's anti-inflammatory effect is due primarily to the presence of hydroxytyrosol and oleocanthals, which are potent painkillers. They also give good olive oil that peppery 'bite' at the back of the throat, which is similar to the taste of aspirin. These chemicals lower the levels of a number of significant markers for inflammation (IL-1, IL-6 and TNFα) and raise nitric oxide (NO).[2] Hydroxytyrosol is also an extremely potent antioxidant, which, among other things, reduces the damage caused to LDL cholesterol.[3] (As we saw earlier, it is difficult to clear damaged LDL cholesterol, which gets dumped in arterial deposits.) Olive oil also seems to aid blood sugar control, as was revealed in a study of type 1 diabetics in which one group was given butter (high saturated fat) while another was given olive oil (high mono-unsaturated fat).[4]

For all these reasons, aim to eat plenty of good-quality olive oil, especially in the high fat phase.

Fats for Fuel

When your reserves of glucose run out, the body can convert fat into either glucose or ketones for energy. In general, saturated fats are best for this, although mono-unsaturated oils can be used for the same purpose.

Short chain fatty acids – such as butyric acid – are found in dairy products sourced from grass-fed animals. Butyric acid, in particular, has significant anti-inflammatory effects in the gut, so it is generally good for gut health. Moreover, a number of animal studies have found that it can reverse insulin resistance.[5] A great source of these chemicals is organic ghee – clarified butter – which contains nothing but fat. Therefore, many people who are unable to tolerate dairy protein can tolerate organic ghee. (The 'organic' part is important because fat-based toxins, including pesticide and herbicide residues, which accumulate in fat, are extremely harmful.) The same is true of goat's cheese, another good source of butyric acid.

Long chain fatty acids – such as myristic acid, palmitic acid and stearic acid – which are prevalent in meat products, tend to raise 'bad' LDL cholesterol. For instance, one study found that excessive amounts of palmitic acid, especially in the absence of linoleic acid, increased blood cholesterol levels.[6] Both palm oil and coconut oil are good sources of linoleic acid, so either may be used to provide protection from the potentially harmful effects of palmitic oil. However, palm oil has a deservedly poor reputation because its cultivation has had a devastating impact on the world's rainforests. This is one of the reasons why we prefer coconut oil. It is also a much better source of beneficial MCTs.

Medium chain fatty acids – such as caproic, caprylic, capric and lauric acids, which are known collectively as MCTs – are found in high concentrations in both coconut oil and dairy butter and convert readily into ketones in the liver. Caproic acid has six chains of triglycerides, caprylic acid eight chains, capric acid ten chains and lauric acid twelve chains, which means it is not far from saturated fat (eighteen chains). A BBC trial split volunteers into coconut oil, olive oil and butter groups, then measured their levels of 'good' HDL and 'bad' LDL cholesterol.[7] Those eating coconut oil saw their LDL decrease and their HDL increase (by 15 per cent). Those in the olive oil group experienced slight reductions in their LDL and slight increases in their HDL. Those eating butter recorded slight increases in both.

Such studies leave little doubt about the health benefits of coconut oil (especially in relation to cardiovascular disease), yet it is 90 per cent saturated fat, 8 per cent mono-unsaturated and only 2 per cent poly-unsaturated – proportions that many people would assume were unhealthy. Palm nut oil is similar, but lower in saturated fat and higher in mono-unsaturates – 81 per cent, 17 per and 3 per cent, respectively. Palm fruit oil is 50 per cent, 40 per cent and 10 per cent, while olive oil is 14 per cent, 73 per cent and 13 per cent. All of these oils are good sources of fuel, and all have their own individual health benefits.[8] For instance, researchers are currently exploring whether MCTs might provide extra protection against epilepsy and Alzheimer's disease, in addition to being good raw material for conversion into ketones.[9]

Going Nuts

Nuts contain saturated, mono-unsaturated and poly-unsaturated fats, but they are predominantly mono-unsaturated. Walnuts have the highest concentrations of omega-3s. All nuts are good sources of protein (with almonds the best), and all contain relatively small amounts of carbohydrates, averaging just 4g in a 28g serving, except for cashews and pistachios, both of which have double this amount. They are all also extremely low GL, with a handful of nuts probably less than 1 GL.

The table overleaf shows the fats in a 28g (1oz) portion of a variety of nuts or a tablespoon of nut butter or oil. Aim to eat at least one or two of these portions each day, not only for their fat content, but also because they are high in protein and polyphenols (as we explain in subsequent chapters). One study has found that intake of nuts and seeds is closely associated with good health, even more so than the consumption of vegetables.[10]

Avoid Trans Fats

As mentioned above, hydrogenated and other trans fats look like the real thing but have none of the health benefits of fats in their original form. They are usually created by high heat, such as frying, and the more unsaturated a fat, the more damage it suffers through exposure to high temperatures. Consequently, never fry with flax seed oil; use butter, lard, olive oil or coconut butter instead. Even better, avoid deep frying altogether by sautéing then steam frying, and certainly never heat oil to the 'smoke point'. Literally millions of harmful oxidants are created when oil starts smoking. This is why barbecuing, especially when fat is allowed to drip onto the hot coals, is really bad news, as is wok frying with sunflower oil. Butter, olive oil and coconut oil all have similar smoke points – 160–177°C. The highest smoke point of the

Type of nut/ nut product	Approx. number	Calories	Protein (g)	Total fat (g)	Saturated (g)	Mono- unsaturated (g)	Poly- unsaturated (g)	Carbs (g)	Fibre (g)
Almond butter	Tbsp	232	9	20	1.6	12	5	2.3	4.2
Macadamia	11	200	2	22	3.5	17	0.5	4	2
Pecan	19 (halves)	200	3	20	2	12	6	4	3
Pine	165	190	4	20	1.5	5.5	10	4	1
Brazil	6	190	4	19	4	7	6	3	2
Walnut	14 (halves)	190	4	18	1.5	2.5	13	4	2
Pistachio	49	160	4	18	1.5	7	4	8	3
Peanut butter (no sugar)	Tbsp	222.5	9	17.5	2.5	9	6	5.7	3
Hazelnut	21	180	4	17	1.5	13	2	5	3
Tahini	Tbsp	235	9.6	20	3.3	6	7	0.7	3.5
Almond	23	160	6	14	1	9	3.5	6	4
Peanut	One-third of a small packet	165	6.6	14	2	7	4.4	1.6	2.4
Cashew	18	160	4	13	3	8	2	9	1

healthier oils is ghee's, at 252°C. (The smoke point of avocado oil is similar, but unfortunately it is not readily available.)

All trans fats have inflammatory properties, whereas raw meat does not, so it seems to be the cooking process that causes the problems, rather than the food itself. However, studies of meat's links to illnesses such as diabetes, heart disease and cancer rarely, if ever, differentiate between its effects in its raw and cooked states.

MCT Oil and Synthetic Ketones

As mentioned in Chapter 5, there are three types of ketones: ace-toacetate (AcAc), beta-hydroxybutyrate (BHB) and acetone (AC). Synthetic ketone esters are the most concentrated source, followed by ketone salts, both of which provide BHB. The former can be obtained in the United States in 25ml 'shots' (see Resources). They still have a number of bureaucratic hurdles to clear in the European Union and the UK, but they should be available in both markets within the next few years. A single 25ml shot rapidly raises the ketone level by 3–4μM, while a 10ml shot (just under half a bottle) increases it by about 1μM.[11] Ketone salts, which are also available in the United States, come in powder form. A 25g scoop raises the ketone level by 0.9μM. Both of these supplements are known as *exogenous* ketones, because you take them into your body from the outside. By contrast, you manufacture *endogenous* ketones from your own reserves of body fat.

The next-best supplemental source of ketones is MCT oil that contains caproic acid (C6), caprylic acid (C8) and/or capric acid (C10) – all of which are medium chain triglycerides (see above). Other MCT oils are derived from lauric acid (C12), but these are less effective. All of these products are manufactured from con-centrated coconut oil. After ingestion, the liver has to convert them into ketones, which means that they have a less immediate effect on blood ketone level than synthetic ketones. Nevertheless, the recommended dose can still replicate levels that are achieved after two to four days of fasting or two days on a very low carb diet. The best MCT oils contain caprylic acid – generally known by the abbreviation C8 – which is transported straight to the liver for conversion into ketones.[12] These raise blood ketone levels by 20–30 per cent more than most mixed MCT oils. (Please note: you must use an oil that contains caprylic acid triglyceride. Capsules of pure caprylic acid are used in the treatment of candidiasis, but they are not suitable for generating ketones.) We prefer C8 oils derived from coconut oil to those from palm oil, for environmental reasons.

The liver converts about half of these MCTs into ketones, while the brain is also able to use roughly a fifth immediately as fuel.[13] One to three tablespoons of C8 oil can raise the blood ketone level by 0.5–1µM and thus give you an instant fuel boost.

The brain functions better when it receives a regular supply of ketones, especially if you are exhausted, about to undertake strenuous exercise, or midway through a marathon. Indeed, as we have seen, neurons tend to prefer ketones to glucose, given the choice. However, although taking synthetic ketones or C8 oil will increase the level of ketones in your blood and so put you in a state of ketosis, it will not initiate ketogenesis, so your body will not start converting its own fat into ketones. To enter that fat burning mode, you must either fast or follow a high fat, low carb diet for at least a couple of days. Supplementing ketones on a daily basis will speed up this process, though.

Good Fats to Eat

We have compiled a list of the best fats to include in your diet, especially during the high fat phase of the Hybrid Diet. (Those that are suitable for vegans are marked with an asterisk.)

- Seeds and nuts, such as flax seeds, chia seeds, pumpkin seeds, pecans, Brazils, macadamias, walnuts and their oils*

- Tahini*

- Olive oil*

- Coconut butter and/or oil*

- Organic ghee or butter

- Cacao butter*

- Palm oil (ideally palm fruit oil)*

- Goat's or sheep's cheese, Brie and hard cheese

- Lard, duck or chicken fat

- Eggs

- Oily fish, such as mackerel, herring, kippers, sardines, salmon, trout and fresh tuna

You will need to eat quite substantial amounts of these foods during the high fat phase, as you're aiming for 15 to 20 per cent of calories from protein, approximately 10 per cent from carbohydrate and 65 to 75 per cent from fat. A good, balanced daily menu for a pescatarian would be: egg and goat's cheese omelette made with organic ghee (breakfast), a serving of oily fish with an avocado and olive oil salad plus a side of spinach sautéed in coconut butter (lunch) and a small serving of a low GL bean dish with a tahini-based sauce (dinner), plus a couple of handfuls of nuts for snacks throughout the day. Ideally, eat five servings of oily fish a week – so lots of smoked salmon, sardines, mackerel, herrings and kippers – as well as plenty of nuts and avocados. These foods have several proven health advantages. For instance, a meta-analysis of twenty studies reported that eating 28g of nuts a day reduced the risk of cancer by 15 per cent.[14] Similarly, an Icelandic study found that women who consumed four servings of fish a week early in life halved their risk of developing breast cancer in middle age.[15] Finally, avocados contain a compound called defensin that may encourage breast cancer cells to self-destruct.[16]

If you are more carnivorous by nature, you could have a cooked breakfast of eggs and sausages, then steak for your main meal. However, you will give yourself too much protein if you include another portion of meat, regardless of whether you are in the high fat or the low GL phase. (See Chapter 21 for why this isn't a good idea.) Limit yourself to a maximum of two portions of meat a day, or ideally one portion of meat and one of fish. If you feel hungry, add more fat, not more protein and certainly not more carbs. This could be a hot drink with a spoonful of coconut oil, a tablespoon of C8 MCT oil or even a shot of synthetic ketones (see Resources).

These supplements are also useful if you do not eat meat or fish, as you may find it difficult to enter ketosis through diet alone. There is more advice on how to follow the Hybrid Diet if you are vegan or vegetarian in Chapter 24.

Chapter 20

Fruit and Veg: Common Ground

Whether you are in the high fat or the slow carb phase, roughly half of every meal needs to be made up of vegetables and/or fruit. With the exception of starchy vegetables (see later), which can only be eaten in the slow carb phase, fruit and veg are therefore the backbone of a good diet. We prefer those that are rich in antioxidants, polyphenols or sirtuin activators (see page 198). Some high performers contain all three.

According to Dr Richard Cutler, former Director of the US Government Anti-ageing Research Department, 'The number of antioxidants that you maintain in your body is directly proportional to how long you will live.' Pollution, smoking and eating barbecued or deep-fried foods on a regular basis can all create an increased need for antioxidants. The longest-lived people on earth – including the residents of Okinawa (Japan), Loma Linda (California) and Ovodda (Sardinia) – eat large amounts of antioxidant-rich fresh fruits and vegetables, which reduce cell damage in the body. Out of Okinawa's population of one million people, there were 900 centenarians at the time of writing – four times more than the UK or US average.

Most people know that they should eat at least five portions of fruit and vegetables each day, but the World Health Organisation actually recommends eight to ten servings, primarily because of fruit and veg's proven role in cancer prevention. After reviewing hundreds of studies, the World Cancer Research Fund concluded that carotenoids – antioxidants that are found in fruit and vegetables – are highly protective. Therefore, it is hardly surprising that a high beta-carotene intake is strongly associated with lower mortality.[17] This is consistent with the results of our own 100% Health survey, which found that eating more fruit and veg (up to ten servings a day) is linked to better health. Another major study found that people who eat seven or more servings of fruit and veg a day have 42 per cent lower mortality, due to their reduced susceptibility to diabetes, heart disease and cancer.[18] Fruit and vegetables are also good for your brain: researchers at Oxford University found that people who eat a lot of fruit and veg tend to have better cognition than those who do not.[19]

Simply eating five servings of fruit and veg a day, not smoking, consuming modest amounts of alcohol and keeping physically active can add up to *fourteen years* to your life, according to one long-term study of 20,000 people.[20] Cutting down sugar and fast carbs will help, too, because both of these increase oxidative stress, which is linked to ageing.[21]

Yet, the average adult in the UK eats only 2.8 portions of fruit and veg per day. Even more alarmingly, one study of nineteen to twenty-four-year-olds found that only 4 per cent of the women in the sample group and *none* of the men achieved the five-a-day target.[22] If vegetables fill half your plate at both lunch and dinner, plus a portion of berries (perhaps with breakfast), some vegetable crudités or a smoothie as a snack, and an apple with some nuts, you will be eating about seven a day (although you should avoid the apple in the high fat phase).

The Best Fruit and Veg

Some fruit and veg – such as bananas, dates and raisins – are high in fast release carbs. These are best avoided at all times, and especially during the high fat phase. Of course, in general, the aim is to eat more fruit and veg because of the nutrients they provide, but not if that exposes the body to a sudden influx of sugar. Therefore, always opt for the low GL varieties, which usually have the added benefit of containing lots of fibre. Also, some fruit and veg are good sources of protein and B vitamins, such as folate, which is found in spinach and other green vegetables, whereas others are not. So, which are the best all-rounders?

Anti-ageing Antioxidants

The way to determine the antioxidant power of a food is to gauge its ORAC (oxygen radical absorbency capacity) potential – an objective measure of its ability to deal with the oxidant 'exhaust fumes' of life. Long-lived people tend to consume at least 6,000 ORACs a day, but what does this mean for your daily diet?

Each of the portions listed below equates to 2,000 ORACs, so any three each day will see you hitting that 6,000 target.

- ⅓ tsp ground cinnamon
- ½ tsp dried oregano
- ½ tsp ground tumeric
- 1 heaped tsp mustard
- ⅕ cup blueberries
- Half a pear, grapefruit or plum
- ½ cup blackurrants, raspberries or strawberries
- ½ cup cherries or a shot of Cherry Active concentrate
- 7 walnut halves
- 8 pecan halves
- ¼ cup pistachio nuts
- ½ cup cooked lentils
- 1 cup cooked kidney beans
- ⅓ medium avocado
- ½ cup of sliced red cabbage
- 2 cups of broccoli florets
- 1 medium artichoke or 8 spears of asparagus

- 1 orange or apple

- 4 pieces of dark chocolate
  (70 per cent cocoa solids)

- ⅓ medium glass (150ml/5fl oz)
  red wine

Source: Oxygen Radical Absorbance Capacity of Selected Foods – 2007, US Department of Agriculture

How to Boost Your Antioxidant Intake

In general, the most colourful and flavoursome foods have the highest antioxidant levels. The reds, yellows and oranges of tomatoes and carrots, for example, are due to the presence of beta-carotene. Artichokes have even higher levels, whereas the likes of carrots, peas and spinach are lower. Deep-coloured fruit, such as blueberries, raspberries and strawberries, also have high levels. All of these are particularly rich in powerful antioxidants called anthocyanidins. For instance, a single cup of blueberries provides 9,697 ORACs. You would need to eat eleven bananas to get a similar benefit!

Therefore, not all portions of fruit and vegetables are the same. In the example below, both days contain the recommended five a day, but Day 2 has 8,000 more ORACs than Day 1.

Day 1 Fruit/vegetable portion	ORAC	Day 2 Fruit/vegetable portion	ORAC
⅛ large cantaloupe melon	315	½ pear	2,617
1 kiwi fruit	802	½ cup strawberries	2,683
1 medium carrot (raw)	406	½ avocado	2,899
½ cup green peas (frozen)	432	1 cup broccoli (raw)	1,226
1 cup spinach (raw)	455	4 spears asparagus (boiled)	986
Total	2,410	Total	10,411

Analysis based on Oxygen Radical Absorbance Capacity of Selected Foods – 2007, US Department of Agriculture

Polyphenol power

In recent years, a great deal of research has shown that a group of compounds known as polyphenols are just as important as a plant's antioxidant power, maybe even more so. Polyphenols are highly concentrated in many so-called 'superfoods', such as resveratrol in the skins of red grapes, isoflavones in beans, curcumin in turmeric, cinnamic acid in cinnamon and anthocyanidins in black elderberries and other berries. As this list suggests, they are a very broad group of compounds that plants produce to protect themselves from infection, UV radiation and other perils. We can benefit from these protective properties, too, because polyphenols seem to be able to switch off disease processes and switch on healthy genetic responses.

It is possible to work out a general polyphenol rating for any food, in much the same way as we can calculate an antioxidant rating. Although such calculations are rather crude, they help us to identify the plants that pack the biggest health punch, especially as quite a few polyphenols also act as antioxidants. However, some do not: for example, peppermint is a terrific source of polyphenols but not so remarkable as an antioxidant, whereas basil is the opposite. We have listed some of our favourites below:

- artichoke
- red onion
- broccoli
- asparagus
- spinach
- olives
- beetroot

- avocado
- kale
- blackcurrants
- blueberries
- plums
- blackberries
- raspberries

- strawberries
- cherries
- apples
- chestnuts
- pecans
- almonds
- chia seeds

- flax
- cloves
- oregano
- turmeric
- capers
- mint
- star anise
- sage

- rosemary
- basil
- thyme
- parsley
- lovage
- ginger
- curry powder
- cinnamon

- dark chocolate
- red wine
- coffee
- peppermint tea
- black tea
- green tea

Skinny sirtuins

Some plant compounds also activate sirtuin genes – nicknamed 'skinny' genes because they play a crucial role in the body's ability to burn fat and build muscle (see page 202 for more on this). The first to be identified was the polyphenol resveratrol, which is extracted from red grape skins. Green tea, cocoa powder, turmeric, kale, red onions, olives, parsley and lovage are other good sources of sirtuin activators. Unfortunately, the levels in many common fruits and veg, such as tomatoes, lettuce, kiwi, carrots and cucumber, are relatively low.

Fructose is Fine ... in Small Quantities

Most of the sugar in apples and berries is fructose, whereas dates, grapes and bananas contain much higher quantities of fast release glucose. Fructose is low GL because the body cannot burn it immediately for energy, but the liver can turn it into fat, which encourages insulin resistance, so go easy on it.

The human body can convert just six teaspoons of fructose into glucose in the course of twenty-four hours. A small apple or a conference pear (the harder the better) contains about two teaspoons of fructose as well as about 5g of fibre, much of which is pectin, which further restricts the release of the sugar. Therefore, it is fine to eat the occasional apple or pear during the Hybrid Diet. On the other hand, if you consume fructose without fibre – or if you eat foods that have been sweetened with corn syrup, which is half fructose and half glucose – the ill effects can be profound. In one study, college students were given a measured amount of either glucose or fructose. Those in the fructose group generated ten times as much fat as those in the glucose group.[23] This is because the body finds it very easy to convert fructose into triglycerides, which it stores in fatty tissue.[24] So, even though it is technically low GI, eating lots of fructose will result in weight gain and, ultimately, metabolic syndrome.[25] Therefore, we advise steering clear of all foods and drinks that have been sweetened with fructose. Eat your fruit; don't drink it!

Even better, seek out foods that are high in xylose, such as berries and plums. You can eat a handful of berries every day, including during the high fat phase. The bluer the berry, the better, so blackcurrants, blackberries and blueberries are all great options. In a recent study, one group of overweight, insulin resistant volunteers who were at high risk of diabetes were given a blueberry smoothie every day for six weeks while another group were given a placebo smoothie (which looked and tasted identical). Those who drank the real thing experienced a 22 per cent increase in their insulin sensitivity.[26]

Plums are a great snack, especially if they are eaten with some protein, such as a few almonds or pumpkin seeds, which slows down the release of sugar and therefore lowers the GL. If you prefer prunes (dried plums), make sure they haven't been soaked in sugar.

Xylitol (crystalline xylose) looks and tastes exactly the same as white sugar, but has only a ninth of sugar's GI (or less than half the GI of fructose). Hence, nine teaspoons of xylitol has the same effect on your blood sugar as one teaspoon of regular sugar. It is also highly preferable to any artificial sweetener. So, if you feel you need a sweetener, perhaps for a cake, use a modest amount of xylitol. Note that it has a mild laxative effect – which is why prunes, which also contain xylose, keep you regular – so you should cut down if you start to experience loose bowel movements. Unsweetened prunes and dried berries are the only dried fruits we recommend, and even these need to be eaten in moderation, and only in the low GL, not the high fat, phase of the Hybrid Diet.

Another advantage of using xylitol in place of sugar is that it can help to prevent tooth decay because the bacteria that feed on it are unable to stick to teeth. One study gave a group of infants xylitol syrup two or three times a day for ten months and another group a placebo.[27] The incidence of tooth decay was more than halved in the xylitol group. 'Our results suggest that exposure to xylitol (8 grams per day) in a twice-daily topical oral syrup during primary tooth eruption could prevent up to 70 percent of decayed teeth,' the researchers reported. 'Dividing the 8 grams into three doses did not increase the effectiveness of the treatment. These results provide evidence that xylitol is effective for the prevention of decay in primary teeth of toddlers.'

Avoid Starchy Vegetables

All vegetables – especially those that are green and grow above ground – are good for you. However, some that grow below ground, such as potatoes, parsnips, sweet potatoes, yams and beetroot, are high GL, especially if cooked. The same is true of cooked sweetcorn. Therefore, avoid all of these starchy vegetables in the high fat phase and eat them in small quantities in the slow carb phase.

All of the squashes – including pumpkin, marrow, butternut

squash and courgette – are good alternatives. These are very slow release vegetables, averaging just 3 GL for an 80g serving, so they are great options for the carb portion of any main meal. If you really like them, you could double the serving size and count them as your fruit and veg portion, too. (See Part 5 for recipe ideas.)

In 2007, a group of Chinese researchers reported that adding pumpkin extract to the diet of type 1 diabetic rats promoted the regeneration of beta-cells in the pancreas.[28] Their conclusion was that 'pumpkin extract is potentially a very good product for pre-diabetic persons, as well as those who have already developed diabetes'. They added that, while patients with full-blown diabetes would probably need to continue their insulin injections, pumpkin extract could drastically reduce the amount they needed. This protective effect is thought to be due to high concentrations of both antioxidants and D-chiro-inositol – a molecule that affects insulin activity – in pumpkins. Therefore, whether you are diabetic or not, you are likely to benefit from including lots of squashes in your diet. Try our delicious Spicy Pumpkin and Tofu Soup (page 341) or our Butternut Squash Salad (page 334).

High Fat and High Protein Vegetables

The best vegetables for protein – and for low carbs – are artichokes, spinach, kale, Brussels sprouts, broccoli, cauliflower, beansprouts, mushrooms, peas, green beans, broad beans and runner beans. All of these can be used in a variety of ways, such as Cauliflower Rice (page 325) or kale sautéed in coconut butter or ghee.

The best 'vegetable' for fat – avocado – is actually a fruit. Avocados are exceptionally rich in mono-unsaturated fat as well as a good source of the eye- and brain-friendly antioxidant lutein. In a recent trial, one group of volunteers ate an avocado a day while another had either a medium potato or a cup of chickpeas with an identical number of calories. Those in the avocado group experienced a 25 per cent increase in lutein levels as well as progressive improvements in memory, cognitive processing and attention tests.[29] Avocados also help the body to absorb three to five times more carotenoids from other foods, such as tomatoes or carrots, if they are eaten together.[30]

Fruit and Veg Guidelines

After taking GL, protein content and antioxidant, polyphenol and sirtuin activator levels into account, we have compiled a list of the twelve best fruit and veg all-rounders. However, please don't think of it as definitive because a host of others have their merits, too. Feel free to experiment and find those that work best for you.

	Low GL	Antioxidant	Polyphenol	Sirtuin Activator
Olives	***	***	***	***
Blueberries	***	***	**	***
Kale/spinach	***	**	***	***
Blackcurrants	**	***	**	***
Broccoli	***	**	***	
Artichoke	***	**	***	
Cabbage (red)	***	***	**	
Asparagus	***	**	**	
Onions (red)	**	*	***	***
Avocado	***	**	**	
Apples	**	**	**	**
Beetroot	*	*	***	

- Have a serving of berries or a couple of plums every day.

- Have two servings of vegetables or a large salad with each main meal.

- In the high fat phase, avoid potatoes, parsnips, sweet potatoes, yams, beetroot, sweetcorn, apples, pears and tropical fruits.

- Avoid bananas, grapes, dates and raisins in both phases.

- Minimise consumption of tropical fruits in the slow carb phase.

- Each portion of potatoes, parsnips, sweet potatoes, yams, beetroot or sweetcorn needs to be no more than 7 GLs in the slow carb phase (use the table on page 247 as a guide).

Chapter 21

Don't Exceed Your Protein Needs

In the early days of ketogenic diets, when so many people jumped on the Atkins bandwagon, the advice was simply to cut out carbs and replace them with fat and protein. One of the easiest ways to do this was to eat a lot of fatty meat, eggs and hard cheese, since all of these foods provide nothing but protein and fat. As a method of weight loss, it was carnivore heaven! Almost all ketogenic diets recommend a portion of meat or other animal protein twice a day. However, there is much to recommend eating fish or vegetable protein instead, as we explain below. Moreover, oily fish has the added benefit of providing plenty of omega-3 fats, which are present in much lower quantities in red meat. We have a name for this variation on the traditional ketogenic diet: Fishkins!

In addition, eating too much protein – especially from animal sources rather than fish or vegetables – has some potentially serious consequences in relation to kidney function, cancer risk, raised insulin and accelerated ageing. So, how much protein do you actually need?

Protein consists of amino acids, which are your body's building blocks. Eight of these are considered 'essential', and you need all eight in roughly the right proportions to remain healthy. This is because enzymes, hormones (such as insulin), neurotransmitters (such as dopamine and serotonin), muscles, cells and even the matrix of bone all contain different proteins. Obviously, getting the right amino acids in the right amounts is crucial in early infancy, yet only 7 per cent of the calories in breast milk are in the form of protein. This shows that you don't need to eat a huge amount of protein to increase your muscle mass, and you can certainly get more than enough without ever touching meat. Think of rhinos, which build a ton of muscle on a diet of grasses, leaves and bushes. (A similar misconception is that you need to drink lots of milk to make healthy bones.)

Assuming that you get all eight essential amino acids from the food you eat, ideally protein should make up no more than 10–15 per cent of your total calorific intake (you may get a little more during the high fat phase, but it shouldn't be much more). This is because getting more than a quarter (25 per cent) of your calories from protein may be harmful over the long term (although athletes both need and can tolerate more; see below). To put this into context, a cooked breakfast of sausage, eggs and bacon will provide almost all of your maximum daily allowance, so anyone who eats meat, fish and/or eggs three times a day will far exceed their limit.

The more protein you eat, the harder your kidneys have to work to eliminate nitrogen-rich waste products from your bloodstream. One meta-analysis of thirty studies found that kidney function declines significantly when consumption of protein exceeds 25 per cent of total calorific intake.[31] Poor kidney function is also a common symptom of diabetes.

Your Ideal Protein Needs

A good way to work out your optimal daily protein intake is to aim for 1g of protein for every 1kg of lean body mass (total weight minus body fat). In the UK, the average body fat percentage is 20 per cent for men (the ideal is 15 per cent) and 30 per cent for women (the ideal is 22 per cent). As an example, if you had 25 per cent body fat (and therefore 75 per cent lean body mass) and weighed 64kg (10 stone), your lean body mass would be 48kg (64 × 0.75), so you aim to eat 48g of protein each day – or 16 grams three times a day.

An alternative method is to look at calorific intake. The average man needs about 2,400 calories and the average woman 2,000 calories each day. As mentioned above, we recommend that approximately 10 to 15 per cent of your calories come from protein: that is, 240 to 360 calories for men and 200 to 300 for women. Protein has four calories per gram, so, on this basis, men need 60 grams, and should not exceed about 90g, and women need 50 grams and should not exceed 75g each day.

In practical terms if you aim for 15 grams of protein three times a day, or 25 grams twice a day, you'll have enough. Since protein-rich foods such as meat, fish and eggs are not pure protein, but also contain fat and water, visually this looks like roughly a quarter of what's on your plate. During the high fat phase, if you choose fatty meats, also high in protein, every day you may get a little more but don't exceed 75g of protein a day for women and 90g a day for men, unless you're an endurance or strength athlete.

How Much is 15g of Protein?

All the portions in the following table equate to 15g of protein.

Food	Weight	Serving
Tofu and tempeh	160g (5¾oz)	¾ packet
Soya mince	100g (3½oz)	3 tbsp
Chicken (with skin)	50g (1¾oz)	1 very small breast or thigh
Turkey	50g (1¾oz)	½ small breast
Steak (rib-eye)	100g (3½oz)	small steak
Quorn	120g (4¼oz)	⅓ pack
Salmon and trout	55g (2oz)	very small fillet
Tuna (canned in brine)	50g (1¾oz)	¼ can
Sardines (canned in brine)	75g (2¾oz)	⅔ can
Cod	65g (2¼oz)	very small fillet
Clams	60g (2⅛oz)	¼ can
Prawns	85g (3oz)	6 large prawns
Mackerel	85g (3oz)	medium fillet
Kipper	75g (3oz)	large fillet
Oysters	15	15
Yoghurt (natural full fat)	285g (10oz)	½ large tub
Brie	75g (2¾oz)	1 cup
Cheddar cheese	63g (2¼oz)	small wedge
Cottage cheese	120g (4¼oz)	½ medium tub
Full fat goat's or sheep's cheese	70g (2½oz)	1 cup
Hummus	200g (7oz)	1 small tub
Milk	440ml (15½fl oz)	large glass
Soya milk	415ml (14½fl oz)	large glass
Eggs (boiled)	2	2
Quinoa	125g (4½oz)	large bowl
Baked beans	310g (11oz)	¾ can
Kidney beans	175g (6oz)	⅓ can
Black-eye beans	175g (6oz)	⅓ can
Lentils	165g (5¾oz)	⅓ can
Nuts (mixed)	100g (3½oz)	small packet
Seeds (based on pumpkin)	50g (1¾oz)	½ cup
Peanuts	50g (1¾oz)	½ cup

Too Much Protein Raises Insulin and Increases the Risk of Diabetes

Why is a high protein diet bad for you? Well, for one, it increases levels of insulin and IGF-1 in the blood. (Although it should be noted that the typical high carb, high protein Western diet is even worse in this respect.) These are two hormones that you want to keep relatively low, because high levels are significant risk factors for cancer. As we saw in Chapter 13, insulin and IGF-1 trigger and work in unison with the mTOR network to promote muscle growth and the production of white blood cells, among other crucial processes. However, the body also needs time to rest and repair during autophagy, which can only begin when mTOR is turned off (see Chapter 14). Unsurprisingly, then, an mTOR network that is driven into a perpetual frenzy by too much insulin and IGF-1 accelerates ageing and increases the risk of contracting cancer. Indeed, virtually all cancers are associated with excessive mTOR activity. After one trial, the researchers concluded, 'Longevity and health were optimized when protein was replaced with carbohydrate to limit compensatory feeding for protein and suppress protein intake ... The results suggest that longevity can be extended in ad libitum-fed animals by manipulating the ratio of macronutrients to inhibit mTOR activation.'[32]

Another reason why a high protein diet might promote the secretion of insulin is because it increases acid load in the bloodstream. The body can 'buffer' short-term increases in acid load, but eating a high protein diet over a long period of time stimulates the overproduction of metabolic acids, a process that has been associated with insulin resistance, loss of blood sugar control and increased risk of diabetes.[33] Vegetable proteins, which contain higher proportions of the alkaline minerals calcium, magnesium and potassium, might help to lower acid load.

Animal versus Fish and Vegetable Protein

Animal – rather than fish or vegetable – protein is usually favoured by advocates of the ketogenic approach, but this puts them at a greater risk of diabetes, according to a large study that followed over 100,000 people over the course of several years. More than 15,000 of them went on to develop the condition and the greater their consumption of animal protein, the higher the risk. Indeed, those in the top fifth of animal protein eaters were 13 per cent more likely to become diabetic. Meanwhile, the researchers claimed that 'substituting 5% of energy intake from animal protein for vegetable protein was associated with a 23% reduced risk'.[34] Again, this may be due to the abundance of alkaline minerals in vegetable protein sources, such as lentils, beans, nuts and seeds, which counterbalance the amino acids in these foodstuffs.

However, many of these foods also contain small amounts of low GL carbs, so they rarely feature in traditional ketogenic diets. This seems to be a very blinkered attitude, especially as low carb diets that derive most of their protein from vegetable sources seem to work quite well. Professor David Jenkins – who invented the glycemic index – gave two groups of volunteers a reduced calorie diet.[35] The first group ate a modest amount of slow release carbs coupled with large portions of fat and vegetable protein. The second group ate more carbohydrates and less fat and protein. The first group's diet was also significantly higher in soluble fibre – for instance, they were given oats instead of wheat as well as plenty of vegetables, such as aubergine and okra – and included seeds, nuts and beans, all of which are excellent high protein foods that are known to lower cholesterol and provide plenty of minerals. Both groups lost almost 9lb in the four-week trial, but those on the low carb diet experienced greater reductions in both their total cholesterol and their 'bad' LDL cholesterol levels.

Our only criticism of this approach is that such diets are

deficient in the omega-3 fats that are known to reduce the risk of cardiovascular disease. The addition of oily fish solves this problem.

What is the Best Protein?

As long as you eat all eight of the essential amino acids in the right proportions, your body will be able to make all twenty-three of the amino acids that it requires to manufacture enzymes, hormones, neurotransmitters and structural tissues. This is why you need less high quality protein with the correct amino acid balance (which is found in meat, fish, eggs, milk, quinoa and soya) than lower quality protein (which is found in nuts, seeds, beans and flowering vegetables, such as broccoli). There are, however, a certain amount of amino acids circulating in the blood at all times, so balancing amino acid intake is important over one or two days, rather than in every meal.

In general, we prefer seafood and vegetarian sources of protein, rather than lots of meat. We see no reason to eliminate meat altogether but limit yourself to small quantities and make sure you choose it carefully: for example, opt for organic and/or grass fed, rather than grain fed, in the case of beef.

Red and Processed Meat and Colorectal Cancer

Many studies have reported a link between large quantities of red and processed meat in the diet and various forms of cancer, especially colorectal cancer. By contrast, there is no evidence that white meat, such as chicken, is a risk factor for cancer.

Colorectal (bowel) cancer is now the second most prevalent cancer in the UK: each year, more than 30,000 people are diagnosed with the disease, and around 18,000 die of it. A US study from 2015 reported a decline in colorectal cancer among people aged over fifty, but a significant rise in younger people. As a result, it predicted a 50 per cent increase in incidence by 2020 – and a doubling by 2030 – in twenty to thirty-four-year-olds.[36] However, according to one conservative estimate, incidence could be *reduced* by 60 per cent through simple diet and lifestyle changes.[37] Although between 5 and 10 per cent of sufferers have a genetic predisposition to bowel cancer, there is no doubt that it is linked to diet and lifestyle. Carcinogens in the food we eat, exacerbated by putrefaction (because of poor digestion and constipation) and the presence of bad bacteria in the gut all play a part. The greatest risk factors are eating a diet that is low in fibre and vegetables but high in calories, animal fat and processed or red meat (especially grilled, barbecued or charred), a history of polyps, smoking, excessive alcohol consumption, lack of exercise and prolonged stress. Grilling, charring and especially barbecuing meat produce known carcinogens called HCAs and PAHs, while processed and cured meat contain carcinogenic nitrosamines because of the use of nitrites in the curing process.[38] (Incidentally, vitamin C inhibits the formation of nitrosamines in the gut, so supplementing it might help to mitigate the risk if you find it impossible to give up bacon or ham.) Haem iron, which is found in red but not white meat, is also a carcinogen.

One of Britain's top bowel experts, Roger Leicester, says, 'Bowel cancer is more likely to develop when people eat a lot of animal fat and there is slow-moving transit of food in the gut.' Both the World Cancer Research Fund and the American Institute of Cancer agree that there is a link between red and processed meat and colorectal cancer. For instance, Professor Martin Wiseman, the World Cancer Research Fund's medical and scientific adviser, has written, 'The evidence on processed meat and cancer is clear-cut. The data show that no level of intake can confidently be associated with a lack of risk. Processed meats are often high in salt, which can also increase the risk of high blood pressure and cardiovascular disease.'[39] Other researchers recommend eating only moderate amounts of red meat and little, if any, processed meat.[40] Indeed, the World Health Organisation classifies all processed meats – including bacon, sausages and ham – as carcinogens. Eating fish, on the other hand, seems to reduce the risk of contracting various cancers. However, even seafood and the essential fats it contains can be damaged by charring or barbecuing.

When you do eat meat, we recommend choosing grass- or pasture-fed or free-range animals, rather than corn-fed or intensively reared (e.g. high carb) animals. Organic meat would fit into this category. These animals are usually fitter and healthier, and their fat content is likely to have more essential fats such as omega-3.

A high fibre diet shortens the length of time that food spends in the digestive tract and thereby reduces the body's exposure carcinogens. In other words, we can minimise our risk of developing colorectal cancer by increasing our intake of fibre and reducing our consumption of red meat, which takes longer to digest. We should all be defecating with ease at least once if not twice a day, but few people do. Among those who completed the 100% Health survey, only 17 per cent of respondents reported one satisfactory bowel movement every day, whereas 45 per cent admitted straining.[41] These findings suggest that close to half of the UK's adult population is suffering from some degree of constipation. The problem is even more prevalent in men, with only one in ten having a satisfactory bowel movement each day.

Soluble fibre also fuels the growth of friendly bacteria, which, in turn, protect the colon. One study compared the intakes of fibre, fat and cholesterol among pre-menopausal South Asian vegetarian women and their Caucasian vegetarian and omnivorous counterparts. The researchers found that a high fibre diet reduced the concentration of bile acids in the subjects' faeces, and therefore reduced the risk of developing colorectal cancer.[42]

By contrast, a low fibre, high refined carb diet elevated beta-glucuronidase, an enzyme secreted by toxic bacteria, which can generate carcinogens in the colon.[43] The activity of this enzyme can be measured in a stool test, such as the Comprehensive Digestive Stool Analysis, which a clinical nutritionist can arrange.

Dairy Products and Cancer

Many traditional ketogenic diets advocate almost unlimited consumption of dairy products, but there are good reasons to be cautious. The evolutionary purpose of milk is to stimulate cell growth and help the newborn infant to develop into a fully grown adult. All mammals stop consuming milk as soon as the initial growth phase is over, except for humans.

Milk contains two proteins (whey and casein) and one sugar (lactose). Bacteria eat the lactose and turn it into lactic acid during cheese and yoghurt production, so these products contain higher proportions of protein than milk itself.

Milk helps cells to grow because it not only contains IGF-1 but stimulates the liver to produce more. And, as we have seen, high levels of IGF-1 are strongly associated with increased risk of cancer. According to Professor Jeff Holly, from Bristol University's Faculty of Medicine, 'Those in the top quarter for blood IGF-1 levels have approximately a three- to fourfold increase in risk of breast, prostate or colorectal cancer.' This opinion was confirmed in a Harvard University study of 20,000 men which found that those with the highest levels of IGF-1 had more than four times the risk of developing prostate cancer than those with the lowest levels.[44] Therefore, we recommend avoiding dairy – or greatly reducing your consumption – especially if you already have any of these cancers, not least because there is evidence that it increases the likelihood of recurrence.[45]

It is the casein in dairy products that increases the level of

IGF-1 in the blood, whereas the whey increases the level of insulin.[46] Indeed, although they are relatively low GL, dairy products trigger substantial secretion of insulin. As we saw in Chapter 13, consistently high levels of insulin and IGF-1 are bad for your long-term health.

There seems to be a particularly strong link between dairy intake and prostate cancer. Indeed, according to the National Cancer Institute, all but four of twenty-three studies have found a positive association between the two.[47] The aforementioned Harvard University study found that participants who consumed more than two dairy servings each day had a 34 per cent higher risk of developing prostate cancer than those who consumed few or no dairy products.[48]

Similarly, in 1937, a group of almost 5,000 UK children started to record their dietary habits. Sixty-five years later, analysis of their reports revealed that those with a high dairy intake during childhood had three times the risk of developing colorectal cancer later in life.[49]

For all these reasons, we advise everyone – and especially men – to cut down on the dairy. It's also a good idea to go entirely dairy free on several days each week. High fat cheeses and fully fermented yoghurt are lower in lactose and therefore carbs, so these are preferable to low fat alternatives.

Exercise and Protein

The amount of protein you need depends on the type and amount of exercise you do, and whether your intention is to build muscle. In general, endurance athletes need to eat something like 1.2–1.4g of protein per kilogram of body mass per day whereas strength athletes need 1.2–1.7g of protein per kilogram.[50] (This calculation relates to body mass, not *lean* body mass, assuming athletes are going to be lean, not overweight.)

A 2017 study explored the protein requirements of experienced young male bodybuilders in order to maintain healthy nitrogen balance (protein contains nitrogen, so this is a good way to determine protein need).[51] Now, it should be remembered that elite bodybuilders need to stimulate IGF-1 and activate mTOR because these are essential for building muscle (see Chapter 13), so their protein requirements are much higher than most people's. The researchers found that the participants needed 1.7–2.2g of protein per kilogram of body mass per day. So, a 75kg bodybuilder might need slightly more than 160g of protein each day – more than three times the recommended amount for the average person.

This leads to an obvious question: is bodybuilding healthy? Is it pushing the human body beyond its natural boundaries, or do big muscles equate to good health? Another study found that men who did regular strength or resistance exercise had 40 per cent less risk of developing cancer than those who did not.[52] This may be because resistance training lowers inflammation and improves insulin balance. It also seems to reduce the risk of breast cancer.[53] So, it's a good idea to build and maintain muscle mass. However, most of us are not bodybuilders, so we don't need to consume more protein. Regular resistance exercise and three 15g portions of protein per day are perfectly sufficient.

How to Get Enough – but Not too Much – Protein from Your Diet

- Eat a 15g portion three times a day or a 25g portion twice a day; for guidance, a meat or fish fillet that would fit in the palm of your hand equates to one portion.

- Eat oily fish (mackerel, herring, kippers, salmon, fresh tuna, trout) or taramasalata (made from fish eggs) at least three times a week.

- Eat white fish twice a week.

- Eat six eggs every week (two eggs per portion).

- Eat a portion (120–180g) of beans, lentils, quinoa, tofu, tempeh or natto at least four times a week.

- Eat a very large serving of vegetable protein in the form of broccoli, cauliflower, spinach, runner beans or peas every day.

- Eat a small handful of nuts or seeds – such as chia, pumpkin, pinenuts, pecans, pistachios, peanuts, almonds, Brazils, walnuts or hazelnuts – as a snack most days; avoid cashews and chestnuts, as these have more carbs.

- Limit consumption of red meat to a maximum of three times a week, and always choose meat from organic, healthy, free range and/or grass-fed animals.

- Free range white meat, such as chicken and turkey, is a healthier alternative.

- Limit consumption of all dairy products to a maximum of three times a week, generally minimise milk, and always choose full fat and fully fermented yoghurt and cheese, such as Brie, Manchego or Swiss, although goat's and sheep's cheese are even better; avoid all 'low fat' products, especially cream cheese.

- Minimise (or ideally eliminate) consumption of all processed meat, including ham, bacon and sausages, and choose only healthy, free range products.

- Avoid all heavily processed meat products.

Chapter 22

The High Fat Phase

In the high fat phase of the Hybrid Diet, your focus is to keep carbs to a minimum and eat a high fat diet with sufficient protein. As in the low carb phase (see Chapter 23), half of a typical meal will be fruit and vegetables, although you must limit your fruit intake strictly to berries and maybe the occasional plum, while roughly a quarter will be protein-rich foods.

While, technically, you could eat nothing but meat or fish and vegetables during this phase, the end result would be an unhealthy amount of protein (see Chapter 21) and/or hunger. The healthy way to counteract both is to increase your intake of fat:

- Eat lots of avocados.

- Go heavy with the oil-based salad dressings.

- Add oil, such as tahini, to your vegetables.

- Sauté spinach in coconut oil, ghee or butter.

- Treat yourself to plenty of oily fish, fatty meats and cheeses as well as nuts and nut butters.

- Drink a shake or two each day, such as a Hybrid Latté (see page 305) or a shake made with C8 MCT oil.

- Take a shot of exogenous ketones.

Such a diet flies in the face of some deeply ingrained fat and calorie phobias, but you will find that it leaves you satisfied and never hungry.

The high fat food plate

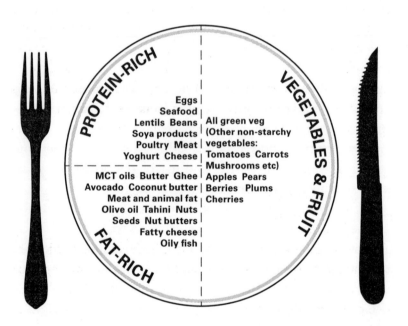

As we saw in Chapter 15, one of the best ways to enter ketosis quickly is through intermittent fasting – not eating for thirteen to sixteen hours each day. For example, on Day 1 (assuming you had dinner at 6 p.m. the previous evening), start the day with nothing but a black coffee or add a dash of full fat milk or cream, a dollop of coconut butter or a tablespoon of C8 oil. The latter is useful if you don't like the taste of coconut, because it has a neutral flavour. Then have breakfast at 10 a.m. and dinner at 6 p.m. This is a relatively easy way to fast for sixteen hours. You could even enhance the effect by substituting a Hybrid Latté (see page 305) for your usual breakfast at 10 a.m., then have lunch at 1 p.m. or whenever you feel hungry. The Hybrid Latté is virtually carb free and rich in MCTs, so it encourages the body to enter ketosis. If you incorporate it into your diet in the way described, you will extend your 'carb fast' to nineteen hours. Not bad for Day 1!

Your body will enter ketosis after another couple of days of this routine, at which point you can switch to thirteen hours of fasting – for example, dinner at 8 p.m. then nothing until breakfast at 9 a.m. Recent technological advances have made it easy to monitor your progress through breath tests, urine sticks or pinpricks of blood. All of these can be used to indicate when you are in and out of ketosis. See Chapter 26 for more details.

The Importance of Low GL in the High Fat Phase

If your goal is to lose weight and burn body fat, you need to eat just enough to stave off hunger (and no more) by limiting your carb intake to 15 GL a day (roughly equivalent to 30g of carbs; see below). While we don't subscribe to the 'calories in, calories out' theory (see page 87), calories are still important. If you eat too many in any form – be it carbs, fat or protein – you will not burn any body fat. On the other hand, if you are in ketosis, your body will meet the vast majority of its energy requirements from its own reserves of fat, which your muscles can burn for energy, and ketones, which it manufactures from fat. It can make the small amounts of glucose it needs from protein. This is one reason why you must include some protein in every meal. Otherwise, your body will start to break down its own muscles to meet its glucose needs.

If your goal is not to lose weight – for instance, if you have adopted the Hybrid Diet to aid your recovery from or alleviate the symptoms of cancer, cardiovascular disease, diabetes, dementia, epilepsy or Parkinson's – there is no specific limit on how much fat you can eat, but do opt for good sources of MCTs, as these generate the most ketones. Use satiation as your guide.

Most ketogenic diets specify a maximum daily amount of 'available' carbs, which might be anything from 10g to 100g. However, you are unlikely to maintain ketosis on 100g of carbs per day unless you do a lot of exercise. Therefore, we advocate a maximum of about 30g a day (see below for more on this).

The 'nutritional information' panel on all food packaging specifies the number of carbs. The illustration below shows the nutritional information that appears on the back of a box of Nairn's rough oatcakes. As you can see, each oatcake provides 6.2g of carbs, so, on the basis of the crude 30g limit, you could eat approximately five a day if they were your only source of carbs. In addition, though, each oatcake contains less than 0.1g sugar, which means that at least 6.1g of those 6.2g are relatively slow carbs. Hence, they have a very low GL rating – 2GLs per oatcake (weighing 10.4g).

Nairn's rough oatcakes nutritional information panel

Ingredients: Wholegrain **oats** (88%), sunflower oil, sustainable palm fruit oil, sea salt, raising agent: sodium bicarbonate.

Nutritional Information

Typical Values	Per Oatcake	Per 100g
Energy	205kJ	1828kJ
	49kal	436kcal
Fat	1.9g	17g
of which saturates	0.4g	3.9g
Carbohydrate	6.2g	55.6g
of which sugars	0.1g	0.8g
Fibre	1.1g	10.1g
Protein	1.2g	10.3g
Salt	0.17g	1.47g
Phosphorus**	39.3mg	350mg
	6% RI	50% RI
Manganese**	0.41mg	3.64mg
	21% RI	182% RI

Reference Intake (RI) of an average intake
(8400kJ/2000kcal)

As the goal is to keep your blood glucose level low, and consequently your insulin level low (which tells your cells to release fat for immediate use as energy or conversion into ketones), and since a food's glycemic load is the best predictor of subsequent blood glucose level, we suggest limiting your carb intake to 15 GL a day, rather than 30g a day. The reason for this is that 30g of white table sugar has a much larger effect on blood glucose and insulin levels than 30g of oatcakes. GL takes this into account. In this example, 30g of sugar has 21 GL, whereas 30g of oatcakes (roughly three) has just 6 GL. (You can find the GLs for a variety of foods at http://gl.patrickholford.com/.) So, while the 30g limit is fine for oatcakes – in fact, you could allow yourself twice this (six oatcakes) – it is far too high for sugar.

By limiting yourself to 15 GL per day, you will ensure that you eat not only low carbs, but slow carbs. On average, this will mean that you will have to eat rather less than 30g of carbs each day (because most foods have a higher GL than oatcakes), so it is a slightly stricter approach. On the other hand, the half a plate of non-starchy vegetables that you have as part of your lunch and dinner are also very low GL. For example, five 100g portions of spinach total just 1 GL. We have assumed that your half a plate of vegetables, twice a day, will give you an average of 4 GL per day, but there's no need to count this as part of your carb allowance: you can still allow yourself 15 GL from other sources. However, it is still a good idea to skew your vegetable choices – or quantities – to the top half of the table below (low GL) and avoid anything in the bottom half (high GL). For example, a medium tomato (70g), has 2 GL – the equivalent of *ten* portions of spinach. So, we advise lots of greens, not so many tomatoes and no potatoes whatsoever.

GL rating	Food	Serving size in g	Looks like	GLs
1	Aubergine E	100	½ small	1
1	Broccoli E	100	1 handful	1
1	Cabbage E	100	1 handful	1
1	Cauliflower E	100	1 handful	1
1	Courgette E	100	1 small	1
1	Cucumber E	100	½ small	1
1	Lettuce E	100	large handful	0–1
1	Radish E	25	1 handful	1
1	Spinach E	100	large handful	1
1	Kale E	75	1 handful	1
1	Avocado E	190	1 medium	1
1	Leeks E	100	1 medium	1
1	Green beans E	75	1 handful	1

GL rating	Food	Serving size in g	Looks like	GLs
1	Tomato E	70	1 medium	2
1	Onion E	180	1 medium	2
1	Asparagus E	125	1 handful	2
1	Carrots	80	1 small	3
1	Green peas	80	1½ tbsp	3
1	Pumpkin/squash	80	1 serving	3
1	Beetroot	80	2 small	5
1	Roasted vegetables	–	1 serving	5
1	Swede	150	⅓ swede	7
1	Sweet potato wedges	–	small serving	8
1	Banana/plantain, green	120	1 very small	8
1	Broad beans	80	2 tbsp	9
1	Sweet potato and carrot mash	–	1 serving	10
2	Parsnips	80	1 medium	12
2	Sweetcorn, on the cob, boiled	150	third of a cob of corn	14
2	Yam	150	1 medium	13
2	Boiled potato	150	3 small	14
2	Microwaved potato	150	3 small	14
3	Mashed potato	150	3 tsp	15
3	New potato, unpeeled and boiled 20 min.	150	3 small	16
3	Instant mashed potato	150	3 tbsp	17
3	Sweet potato	150	1 large	17
3	Baked potato, white, baked in skin	150	1 large	18
3	French fries	150	20	22

All vegetables marked E have an estimated GL score.

Another way to lower the GL of your meals is always to eat carbs with protein and fat, never on their own. For example, eating two scrambled eggs with an avocado and an oatcake will lower the GL of the whole meal by about 20 per cent. So that 2 GL oatcake becomes the equivalent of a 1.6 GL oatcake.

Finally, there is one more trick – glucomannan fibre. If you take 1g (half a teaspoon or two capsules) at the start of every meal (always with a large glass of water), you will lower the GL of that meal by a further 20 per cent. So the 1.6 GL oatcake now has the equivalent effect of 1.3 GLs! Glucomannan fibre has an added benefit, too. One of the drawbacks of a high fat diet can be constipation, whereas too much MCT oil can make bowel movements quite loose. Glucomannan bulks up faecal matter, making it easier to pass. Experiment to find the dosage that works best for you.

As we explain in the next chapter, when you switch to the slow carb phase of the Hybrid Diet, you should triple your limit to 45 GLs a day but keep your calorific intake much the same by eating less fat. This will enable you to continue to lose weight without feeling hungry and might even reverse diabetes. However, your body will not be in ketosis so autophagy will not be triggered.

If you don't need to be in ketosis but would like to kickstart weight loss, you have the option of doubling your daily GL limit to 30 GLs while still eating high fat or perhaps drinking a keto-friendly shake each day. This halfway house is worth exploring, but overall we think that the better option is to switch regularly between the high fat and slow carb phases.

Beware of Meat Protein

As we saw in Chapter 21, eating excessive amounts of protein over a long period of time has been linked to a variety of health problems. However, you don't need to worry about this if you follow our recommendations for the Hybrid Diet. Even in the high fat phase, your protein intake will remain optimal – or only marginally higher – as long as you are careful. Moreover, we recommend remaining in that phase for no more than one week a month after your first period of ketosis.

In terms of calories, you will probably eat about 15 to 20 per cent in protein form, around 10 per cent as carbohydrates and 70 to 75 per cent as fat. However, please don't think that you need to conduct a full nutritional analysis of everything you intend to eat and then get the calculator out. The Hybrid Diet is much simpler than that.

In practical terms, once you have filled half of your plate with vegetables and a quarter with protein, you simply add good sources of fat to the point where you are no longer hungry. The fat could comprise the main part of the meal – such as a fillet of mackerel – but often it is 'invisible' because it is added to the vegetable or protein portion, such as olive oil, tahini and nuts in an avocado salad, or coconut oil in sautéed vegetables.

More Fish, Less Meat

Aim to eat at least 20g of protein twice a day (see Chapter 21), although it is fine for each of these meals to contain more like 30g during the high fat phase (that is, two of the portions listed in the table on page 207). The 'protein' quadrant of your plate will provide 15g, while the remaining 5g might come, for instance, from a combination of starchy and low GL vegetables in the 'fruit and vegetable' sector.

Below we list all of the 15g portions of seafood and meat from the table on page 207. As we explained in Chapter 17, fish has much higher concentrations of essential omega-3 fats and a number of other health benefits, but this does not mean that you should never touch red meat again. Rather, try to limit yourself to a maximum of three portions of organic meat from grass-fed animals each week and aim to get the majority of your protein from seafood, and especially oily fish. It's also a good idea to choose fattier meat, including the skin, in the high fat phase. All of the higher fat options are marked with an asterisk.

Food	Weight	Serving
Chicken (with skin)*	50g (1¾oz)	1 very small breast or thigh
Turkey	50g (1¾oz)	½ small breast
Steak (rib-eye)*	100g (3½oz)	small steak
Quorn	120g (4¼oz)	⅓ pack
Salmon and trout	55g (2oz)	very small fillet
Tuna (canned in brine)	50g (1¾oz)	¼ can
Sardines (canned in brine)	75g (2¾oz)	⅔ can
Cod	65g (2¼oz)	very small fillet
Clams	60g (2⅛oz)	¼ can
Prawns	85g (3oz)	6 large prawns
Mackerel*	85g (3oz)	medium fillet
Kipper*	75g (3oz)	large fillet
Oysters	15	15

Fat Units

As the name suggests, you can eat liberal amounts of fat every day during the high fat phase. If you eat 2,000 calories a day – the recommended daily amount for women – then at least 1,300 of those calories (65 per cent) should come from fat. A tablespoon of tahini or peanut butter, or a flat tablespoon of oil, is about 150 calories. So, 1,300 calories is in the region of 9 tablespoons (or three tablespoons, three times a day).

We have invented a unit of measurement called the Fat Unit (FU), which equates to 130 calories from fat, so women should aim for ten of these a day during the high fat phase. For instance, you could eat 3 FUs at each of your three main meals and 1 FU in a snack. Alternatively, if you have three tablespoons of C8 MCT oil each day (the fastest way to enter ketosis), you could have just 2 FUs at each meal and 1 FU in a snack. You could also skip the snack (and therefore reduce your total intake of calories) if your aim is to lose weight.

Our Hybrid Latté, which is roughly 400 calories and provides almost 20g of protein, is 3 FUs (see page 305). So, nothing but three of these per day would give you sufficient protein to meet your body's needs, about 9 FUs and 1,800 calories.

The table below lists foods with high concentrations of MCTs. It's a good idea to focus on these during the high fat phase.

Food	Calories	Serving	Fat
Hybrid Latté	429	1 glass	3
C8 MCT oil	155	1 tablespoon	1
Coconut oil	117	1 tablespoon	1 –
Nuts and seeds	143	small handful	1
Nut butter	150	1 tablespoon	1 +
Tahini	150	1 tablespoon	1 +
Oily fish	50	1 fillet	½
Taramasalata	207	½ a 170g tub	2 –
Avocado	250	1	2
Butter/ghee	115	20g	1
Creamy goat's cheese	140	50g	1
Cheddar	180	60g	1 +
Brie	146	60g	1 +
Coconut yoghurt (Coconut Collective)	103	small tub (125g)	1
Coconut yoghurt (Rebel Kitchen)	139	200g	1
Chicken thigh	140	100g	1

Food	Calories	Serving	Fat
Rib-eye steak	200	100g	1½
Pork chop	84	1 (85g)	½
Sausage	140	1 (50g)	1
Eggs	94	2	1 –
Bacon, pork or salmon	190	2 slices	1½

(+/- means a little bit higher or lower than number given)

If you have two scrambled eggs (1 FU), a slice of smoked salmon (¾ FU) and half an avocado (1 FU) with a rough oat-cake for breakfast, you will be just short of the suggested 3 FUs per meal.

For lunch, you could have some chicken thigh, a pork chop or a sausage (all 1 FU) with half a plate of spinach or kale sautéed in two tablespoons of coconut oil, butter or ghee (2 FUs). If you went for a mackerel fillet instead of the meat, the meal would be 2½ rather than 3 FUs.

In the afternoon, you could have a Hybrid Latté, which includes a tablespoon of C8 MCT oil, a heaped tablespoon of nut butter and a handful of nuts in carb free almond milk (3 FUs). Alternatively, as a snack, you could dip celery sticks in half a pot of taramasalata with 100g of goat's cheese (2 FUs), or opt for a smaller (1 FU) portion.

In the evening, you could go vegetarian if you feel you've already had enough meat or fish and protein for the day. How about a chilli made with beans and vegetables, all sautéed in a tablespoon of olive oil, with a tablespoon of tahini stirred in at the end (2 FUs)? If you grate some Cheddar cheese on top, you will add another FU.

This combination of meals and snacks would give you at least the recommended 10 FUs, very few carbs and enough – but not too much – protein.

In reality, you probably will not want to eat this much,

because fat is very satisfying. If so, skip the snack. Don't worry if you don't always hit the target of 10 FUs, but try to eat a minimum of 8 FUs each day as this will ensure that the majority of your calories come from fat rather than carbs. As mentioned earlier, you could always have one or two tablespoons of C8 MCT oil straight off the spoon if you find it difficult to eat 8 FUs at mealtimes. Alternatively, you could boost your FU intake by starting your day with coffee and a dollop of coconut oil or cream.

You can check the amount of fat that any food contains by looking at the nutritional information panel on the packaging. By law, this has to state the amount of fat per serving in grams. Multiply by nine to get fat calories per serving. So, if one serving contains 10g of fat, that's 90 calories – about three-quarters of an FU. Also check the carbs, because you should be aiming for a maximum of 30g a day.

Bear in mind, though, that this is based on the recommended number of calories – 2,000 per day – for an 'average' woman. If you are an 'average' man, you may need a bit more. If you do a great deal of exercise, you will need a lot more. On the other hand, if you are trying to lose weight, it might be a good idea to aim for fewer total calories (maybe 1,800), with the same proportion (65 per cent) derived from fat. You will raise your ketone levels on a ketogenic diet, but you will not release and burn your reserves of fat if you eat far more calories than your body needs, regardless of whether they come from fat or carbs. So, for weight loss in the high fat phase, eat as much fat as you need to stave off hunger, but no more than that.

Limit Your Carbs

Most of the meal options listed above contain almost no carbs. This is quite a good principle to follow when you're getting started and switching your metabolism to running on ketones. However, once you've made the switch, you can allow yourself a few more carbs, ideally spread throughout the day.

You'll learn much more about carbs in the next chapter, but below we give a short list of the best carb foods to eat (in moderation) during the high fat phase. All of the following provide about 5 GL of slow release carbs, so you can allow yourself about three per day:

- A small bowl of strawberries, raspberries or blueberries

- Half an apple

- A plum

- Two oatcakes (choose rough and/or organic)

- A thin slice of pumpernickel bread

- A cup of oats

- A small serving (135g) of Kamut bulgur (half a cup dry weight – 45g)

- A small serving of squash (130g)

- A small carrot (115g)

- A small serving of swede (107g)

- A small serving of (90g) quinoa (third of a cup dry weight – 30g)

- Half a small sweet potato

- Two small boiled potatoes

- A 90g packet of peanuts

The Meat and Dairy Free High Fat Phase

If you are vegetarian, you will probably eat plenty of eggs, cheese, avocados, coconut-based products (including C8 oil), nuts, seeds, nut butters and tahini during the high fat phase. However, there are carbs in many vegetarian foods, so do always read the labels carefully. For instance, Rebel Kitchen's and Coconut Collective's coconut yoghurts are both excellent sources of fat, but the former contains only 0.8g carbs per 125g serving, whereas a 120g pot of the latter delivers a whopping 7g.

If you are a dairy free pescatarian, you will obviously eat quite a lot of fish, and possibly a couple of pots of taramasalata each week, as well as avocados, coconut-based products (including C8 oil), nuts, seeds, nut butters and tahini.

Sample Menus

Below, we suggest five days of menus to get you started in the high fat phase. (All of the recipes are in Part 5.) We provide the FU and the GL calculations for each meal, and you will see that all of the food adds up to approximately 10 FUs and a maximum of 15 GLs each day. You will probably find that one snack per day is enough, or you could skip them altogether as you become 'fat adapted' by eating a substantial breakfast, lunch and dinner. Also note that all of the menus provide a safe and healthy daily amount of protein and offer meat, fish and vegetarian alternatives.

We've incorporated suggested mealtimes and intermittent fasting advice to help you kickstart your transition into ketosis in the first two days.

Patrick ate the Day 1, 2 and 3 menus and measured his glucose and ketone levels throughout those three days. The results are on page 296.

Day 1

Finished dinner by 7 p.m. the previous evening.

7 a.m.   Coffee with a dollop of coconut butter or tbsp of Ketofast (C8 oil), or neat C8 oil **1 FU 0 GL**

10 a.m.   2 egg omelette with smoked salmon and avocado **2.5 FU 2 GL**
(After 15 hours of intermittent fasting with no carbs)

1 p.m.   Hybrid Latté (includes 1 tbsp C8 oil) **3 FU 3 GL**

4 p.m.   Half a tub of taramasalata with celery or cucumber sticks **2 FU 1 GL**

7 p.m.   Vegetarian Chilli with tahini or Chilli con Carne, plus 1 tbsp C8 oil **1.5 FU 6 GL**
Total: 10 FU 12 GL

Day 2

7 a.m.   Coffee with a dollop of coconut butter or tbsp of Ketofast (C8 oil); if this isn't sweet enough, add half a teaspoon of xylitol (0.2 GL) **1 FU 0 GL**

10 a.m.   Coconut yoghurt, berries and walnuts **2 FU 2 GL**
(After 15 hours of intermittent fasting with no carbs)

1 p.m.   Marinated salmon steak or chicken thigh with sautéed kale and spinach **2 FU 1 GL**

4 p.m.   Caffeine free Hybrid Latté **3 FU 3 GL**

7 p.m.   Tuna steak with salad, including vinaigrette, green beans and olive oil **2 FU 3 GL**, or Chicken Curry (**2 FU 9 GL**), or Cauliflower, Chickpea and Egg Curry (**2 FU 9 GL**)
Total (maximum): 10 FU 15 GL

Day 3

Breakfast 3 slices of bacon, or smoked salmon, with 2 scrambled eggs **3 FU 0 GL**

Lunch Peruvian Quinoa Salad **2 FU 8 GL**

Snack Goat's cheese with a handful of nuts **2 FU 1 GL**, plus 1 tbsp C8 oil **1 FU 0 GL**

Dinner Low Carb Kedgeree **2 FU 4 GL**
Total: 10 FU 13 GL

Day 4

Breakfast Hybrid Latté **3 FU 0 GL**

Snack ½ avocado with ½ tbsp of tahini **1½ FU 0 GL**, or guacamole with celery or cucumber sticks **1½ FU 2 GL**

Lunch Baked salmon or hot smoked salmon with crème fraîche and herb sauce, with spinach or kale sautéed in ghee or coconut oil and pesto **2 FU 4 GL**

Snack Goat's Cheese and Artichoke Paté, or Hummus and Egg Paté with crudités **1 FU 4 GL** (you may well skip this if not feeling too hungry), plus 1 tbsp C8 oil **1 FU 0 GL**

Dinner Bangers and Cauliflower Mash **2 FU 5 GL**
Total (maximum): 9½ FU 15 GL

Day 5

Breakfast Salmon with Asparagus Omelette **1 FU 0 GL**, plus 1 tbsp C8 oil **1 FU 0 GL**

Snack ½ avocado with ½ tbsp tahini **1½ FU 0 GL**

Lunch Hummus Soufflé **½ FU 5 GL**, plus 1 tbsp C8 oil **1 FU 0 GL**

Snack Gravadlax with Quail's Eggs **1 FU 0 GL**

Dinner   Spiced Turkey Burgers, or Nick's Beefburgers, or
            Rib-eye Steak with Cauliflower Mash **1–2 FU 3 GL**,
            plus 1 tbsp C8 oil **1 FU 0 GL**
            Total (maximum): 9 FU 8 GL

Chapter 23

The Slow Carb Phase

The key factor to remember in the slow carb phase is the glycemic load (GL) of the carbs you eat. Neither fat nor protein substantially affects blood sugar, but carbs do, so you need to prioritise slow carbs, which are low GL, to optimise your health, weight and energy.

In visual terms, half of your plate will comprise vegetables and/or low GL fruit, one-quarter protein-rich foods and one-quarter carbohydrate-rich foods (see overleaf). If you prefer to think in terms of calories, this equates to around 15 to 20 per cent of your total calorific intake from protein, 30 to 35 per cent from fat and 50 per cent from slow carbohydrates. Our focus is not on fats in this phase, but there is no need to avoid the healthy fats in nuts and seeds, their oils and oily fish.

Slow carb food plate

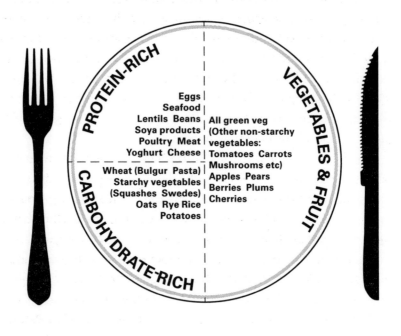

PROTEIN-RICH

VEGETABLES & FRUIT

CARBOHYDRATE-RICH

Eggs
Seafood
Lentils Beans
Soya products
Poultry Meat
Yoghurt Cheese

All green veg
(Other non-starchy
vegetables:
Tomatoes Carrots
Mushrooms etc)
Apples Pears
Berries Plums
Cherries

Wheat (Bulgur Pasta)
Starchy vegetables
(Squashes Swedes)
Oats Rye Rice
Potatoes

In the slow carb phase, aim for 45 GL a day, distributed evenly throughout the day: 10 GL in each of the three main meals, two 5 GL snacks (mid-morning and late afternoon), plus an additional 5 GL for drinks and/or desserts. So, you will be able to have a low GL dessert, diluted fruit juice or even a small glass of dry white wine or spirit.

What to Eat for Breakfast

When you wake up, your blood sugar is low because you haven't eaten for hours, so you need to give your body some fuel (unless you're purposely fasting). During the high fat phase this can be fat, as in the Hybrid latté; in the slow carb phase opt for a low GL breakfast such as eggs with oatcakes or Scandinavian-style rye bread.

Some people think that they'll eat less and lose weight if they avoid eating throughout the morning. However, this idea has been put to the test. One group of volunteers ate three meals and two snacks at the traditional times, while another ate exactly the same food between noon and 11 p.m. The delayed eaters gained more weight and had less healthy metabolism.[54] Another study found that establishing a routine in which you eat at regular intervals throughout the daylight hours allows your metabolism to adjust and provide all the energy you need.[55]

So, if you struggle with fluctuating energy levels and tend to fall asleep during the day, or find it difficult to lose weight, switch to our daily regime of three meals and two snacks. This will help you to avoid an all too familiar scenario: you try to prop yourself up with liquid stimulants (coffee or tea), nicotine, or instant sugar in the form of a piece of toast or a croissant, but the resolve to go without food still weakens as your blood sugar dips lower and lower. Finally, you buckle under the strain and end up bingeing on high GL foods.

This is why you must eat a healthy breakfast. But *what* should you eat and *how much*? Nutritionists gave one group of children a low GL breakfast and another group a high GL breakfast, then allowed both groups free access to a buffet lunch. Although both groups declared that they were satisfied immediately after breakfast, at lunchtime the high GL group were hungrier and ate more food.[56] Another study reported exactly the same result in adults.[57]

The message is clear: eat a low GL breakfast. It will satisfy you for longer by keeping your blood sugar more stable, so you will eat less later. There are two ways to do this:

1. Simply choose any of the low GL breakfasts on pages 329–333. Each of these gives you sufficient protein and essential fats but no more than 10 GL of carbs.

2. Alternatively, 'do it yourself', using the illustration below as a guide.

Slow carb breakfast guidelines

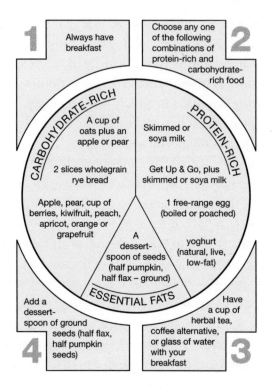

The following breakfasts will give you the perfect balance of carbohydrate and protein:

Carbohydrates	+	Protein
Cereal/fruit	+	Seeds/yoghurt/milk
Fruit	+	Yoghurt/seeds
Fruit	+	Get Up & Go with CarboSlow®/milk
Bread/toast	+	Egg
Bread/toast	+	Fish (such as kippers)

Get Up & Go Breakfasts

One of the simplest and best breakfasts is Get Up & Go – a delicious powder made from a variety of whole foods, including quinoa, oats, seeds, almonds and cinnamon, with lots of added vitamins and minerals, such as vitamin C (939mg per portion), B vitamins and chromium (50mcg per portion), all of which are essential for a healthy metabolism.

It's guaranteed to fill you up until lunchtime, yet each serving is only 283 calories and 5 GLs, so you could blend it with 5 GLs of strawberries, raspberries, pear or blackcurrants for a healthy, balanced breakfast. A teaspoon of cinnamon will make this shake extra tasty. Alternatively, add a scoop of Get Up & Go to two cups of milk or carb free almond milk and a handful of berries. (Tip: frozen berries defrost almost instantly in a blender.)

An even better, even lower GL version is Get Up & Go with CarboSlow®, which includes 1g of super-soluble glucomannan fibre in each serving. Or you can buy CarboSlow separately and add it to original Get Up & Go yourself (see Resources). A serving of Get Up & Go with CarboSlow plus berries and carb free almond milk is just 7 GLs (or 9 GLs if you use oat milk), so you could even make it your regular breakfast in the high fat phase, especially if you add some C8 oil. Equally, because it is perfectly balanced for protein, carbs, vitamins and minerals, you could simply drink a glass three times a day during the slow carb phase, which would see you cruising along on a mere 21 GLs (well below your 45 GLs allowance). However, this would leave you deficient in omega-3 fats, so we would recommend adding a dessertspoon of chia seeds and/or a fish oil supplement.

Cereal Breakfasts

If you prefer a more traditional cereal-, fruit- or toast-based breakfast, there are a few points to consider.

First, any cereal-based breakfast must comprise a low GL cereal and low GL fruit as a sweetener, plus sufficient protein and essential fats. Remember, the goal is no more than 10 GL.

Each of the portions in the table below provides 5 GL. As you can see, the best 'value', in terms of satisfying your hunger, are oat flakes, either cooked (as in porridge) or eaten raw (like cornflakes). Basically, you can eat as much as you like, given that two servings will fill up anybody.

Cereal	Serving size
Oat flakes	2 servings or cups
All-Bran	1 serving (½ bowl or 1 cup)
Unsweetened muesli	1 small serving (less than ½ bowl or ¾ cup)
Alpen	½ serving (¼ bowl or ½ cup)
Raisin Bran	½ serving (¼ bowl or ½ cup)
Weetabix	1 biscuit

Tip: Adding a spoonful of oat bran will lower the GL of any cereal.

Obviously, these cereals can be quite dull on their own, so you might want to consider adding fruit. Again, each of the portions in the table below is equivalent to 5 GL.

Fruit	Serving size
Berries	1 large punnet
Pear	1
Grapefruit	1
Apple	1 small (fits in the palm of your hand)
Peach	1 small
Banana	Less than half

So, to keep hunger at bay, your best option would be porridge (or raw oat flakes) with as many berries as you could eat. Alternatively, you could have half a bowl of All-Bran and a grapefruit, or half a bowl of unsweetened muesli with a small apple.

As far as protein is concerned, there is some in both milk and soya milk (but always pick the unsweetened kind). Rice milk is high GL so best avoided. Oat milk is not bad, but not as good as soya. Yoghurt (unsweetened and well fermented, which gives it a bitter taste) is roughly the same as milk or soya milk, so feel free to have a spoonful on your cereal.

Seeds are another good source of protein, and they also contain countless vitamins, minerals, essential fats and fibre. So, we recommend a tablespoon of ground seeds on your cereal. Ground chia seeds are the best choice because they are high in both protein and soluble fibre. Also, you don't have to grind them because they have a soft outer husk. If you leave your cereal and chia for a few minutes, the seeds will soften and be less crunchy when you eat them. Flax seeds are the next best option, but not as tasty. Pumpkin seeds are good, too, and high in magnesium.

The best cereal-based breakfast is Low GL Granola, which is made by mixing oat flakes with Lizi's Low GL Granola, ground seeds and fresh berries (see page 331). One serving (8 GLs) is completely satisfying.

Yoghurt Breakfasts

If you are especially fond of yoghurt, you could dispense with the cereal and just have yoghurt, fruit and seeds. Each of the following portions provides about 5 GL, assuming that a small pot is 150g:

Yoghurt	Serving size
Plain yoghurt	2 small pots, 300g (11oz)
Non-fat yoghurt	2 small pots, 300g (11oz)
Low fat yoghurt with added fruit and sugar	⅔ small pot, 100g (3½oz)

So, provided you choose a yoghurt that has no added sugar, you can eat two small pots, sweeten it with any of the fruits in the previous table and add a tablespoon of ground seeds. There is absolutely no need to go for the low fat option.

Egg and Toast Breakfasts

Half of the calories in every egg come from fat, but the *type* of fat depends on what the chicken has been fed. For instance, eggs from intensively reared chickens are high in saturated fat. Fortunately, though, most free-range chickens are fed much healthier diets that provide a healthier balance of fatty acids.

Unsurprisingly, omega-3-rich free range or organic eggs are much better for you than ordinary eggs, but we still recommend no more than six of these a week. For example, you could have either two small or one large egg for breakfast every other day. Poach, boil or scramble them, because the high heat of frying damages the essential fats.

As eggs are pure protein and fat (and therefore 0 GL), you could combine them with any of the following, all of which provide 10 GLs of carbs:

Food	Serving size
Oatcakes	4
Pumpernickel	2 thin slices
Sourdough rye bread	2 thin slices
Wholemeal rye bread (yeasted)	1 slice
Wholemeal wheat bread (yeasted)	1 slice

Even high fibre white bread is best avoided, as just one slice would see you exceeding your breakfast allowance of 10 GLs. We recommend oatcakes, Scandinavian-style pumpernickel, sonnenbrot- or volkenbrot-type breads, or yeast-free sourdough rye bread instead. All sourdough breads are substantial, flavoursome and high in fibre. By contrast, light, white, fluffy 'fake' breads are full of air, super-refined and nutritionally inferior. Making the switch to 'real' bread might be a bit of a shock at first, but you'll soon discover that they are much more satisfying as well as healthier.

Real breads are often made from ancient grains, which are genetically simpler than the modern alternatives because they are not the result of decades of hybridisation. The flour is coarsely (stone) ground, which delays the release of sugars and therefore lowers the GL score, and it has far fewer additives than fake flours. An added advantage of sourdough is that it is made without yeast. There is also growing evidence that sourdough fermentation may break down gluten.[58] While the gluten in modern wheat has been widely condemned, ancient wheats, such as kamut bulgur (see page 166), are actually anti-inflammatory, even though they contain gluten. This leads to the inevitable conclusion that something else in modern wheat must be triggering all of those immune reactions. The ill-effects can't be due to gluten alone. There is little or no evidence to support the extreme view that 'all grains are poison'; and, as usual, the plot thickens with every new piece of research.

Moreover, some grains are healthier than others because of the type of carbohydrate they contain. Oats are best, followed by barley and rye. Whereas the GL of wheat varies widely depending on cooking time, oats are much more consistent. Whole oats, rolled oats and oatmeal (which is used to make oatcakes) are all low GL.[59] (Tip: You can lower the GL of porridge by leaving it to cool before eating ... if you happen to like cold porridge!) Pick rough oatcakes as opposed to fine, as these contain more soluble fibre, which reduces the glycemic load. Oat pancakes are another tasty option.

Fishy Breakfasts

Although they have gone out of fashion, kippers (smoked herring) make a tasty and highly nutritious low GL breakfast. Rich in protein and omega-3 fats, a single kipper and any of the bread portions in the previous table will meet all of your protein and fat needs and keep you below the 10 GL target.

What to Eat for Snacks

'Grazing' (eating little and often) is healthier than 'gorging' (eating one or two big meals per day) because it helps to keep your blood sugar even.[60] This makes overeating far less likely, as you will never experience between-meal hunger pangs.

For this reason, we recommend a mid-morning and a late afternoon snack. Each snack should be no more than 5 GL plus some protein, so fruit combined with nuts or seeds is a good option. The fruit portions in the table below all provide 5 GL:

Fruit	Serving size
Strawberries	1 large punnet
Plums	4
Cherries	1 small punnet
Pear	1
Grapefruit	1
Orange	1
Apple	1 small (fits into the palm of your hand)
Peach	1 small
Melon/watermelon	1 slice

Berries – such as raspberries, blueberries and blackberries – plums and cherries are the best 'value' fruit snacks. You can lower the GL of all these fruits by eating them with five almonds or a tablespoon of pumpkin seeds. Almonds have the highest protein to calories ratio of any nut aside from chestnuts. Pumpkin seeds contain even more protein and they are also a good source of omega-3 fats.

'Real' bread (see page 243) and a protein-rich spread such as cottage cheese, hummus or peanut butter is another good snack option. Simply halve the bread servings in the table on page 242 for an indication of 5 GL portions. Hummus tastes especially good with oatcakes, or have it on rye bread or with a raw carrot. (Even a large carrot is less than 5 GLs.) As you have probably gathered, we are big fans of oatcakes, and indeed oats in general, which are great for weight loss and controlling blood sugar.[61] However, avoid any products that contain added sugar. A much better option is a sugar-free, organic oatcake, made with palm fruit oil (unsaturated fat) rather than palm oil (saturated fat). (Try Nairn's brand.) If you like peanut butter, buy the kind with no added sugar. Or you could have sugar-free baked beans on toast.

All of these snacks are 5 GLs:

- A thin slice of rye bread/two oatcakes plus ½ small tub of cottage cheese (150g/5½oz)

- A thin slice of rye bread/two oatcakes plus ⅓ small tub of hummus (100g/3½oz)

- A thin slice of rye bread/two oatcakes and peanut butter

- Crudités (sliced carrot, pepper, cucumber or celery) and hummus

- Crudités and cottage cheese

- A small yoghurt with no added sugar (150g/5½oz) plus berries

- Cottage cheese plus berries

If you would prefer something hot, a satisfying bowl of Chestnut and Butter Bean Soup (page 339) is just 4 GLs.

As you can see, you won't be bored between meals, as there's plenty of scope for mixing and matching.

What to Eat for Lunch and Dinner

But what about those main meals? Well, as you will see in Part 5, we've come up with a host of delicious recipes.

As in the high fat phase, roughly half your plate will consist of very low GL vegetables, such as peas, broccoli, runner beans, courgettes, kale and carrots (in moderation), among many others (see page 222 for the complete list). Remember, you are aiming for a total of 10 GL during lunch or dinner, so this part of your plate should not exceed about 4 GLs. The protein-rich quadrant might include a portion of meat, fish or tofu, while the final carb-rich sector is the place for starchier vegetables, such as parsnips or swedes, and/or grain products, such as pasta and bread. (The latter takes the place of the fat-rich quadrant in the high fat phase.) These two quarters should add up to a maximum of 6–7 GLs.

More Fish, Less Meat

As we saw in Chapter 21, aim to eat at least 20g (⅔oz) of protein – or up to 30g (1oz) in the high fat phase – at both lunch and dinner. The protein-rich part of your plate will meet about three-quarters of this on its own. (See the table on page 207 for the complete list of servings that provide 15g of protein.) Meanwhile, the starchy vegetables in the carb-rich quadrant and the very low GL food in the vegetables quadrant will provide the remaining 5g (⅙oz).

It bears repeating that seafood is a rich source of omega-3 fats, which have proven health benefits, so it is a good idea to get most of your daily protein requirements from fish, rather than meat (and especially non-organic, red meat).

Starchy vegetables

The carb-rich quadrant will usually be about the same size and/or weight as the protein sector, but there can be some variations. For example, if you are eating chicken with rice, the rice portion will look significantly larger than the fillet of chicken because chicken is dense and heavy while rice is relatively light.

Remember, this quarter of the plate accounts for a maximum of 7 GL, so let's see what that means in terms of portion size:

Food	Serving size
Kamut bulgur	Large serving, 190g (7¾oz)
Pumpkin/squash	Large serving, 185g (6¾oz)
Carrot	1 large, 160g (5¾oz)
Swede	Large serving, 150g (5½oz)
Quinoa	Large serving, 130g (4½oz)
Beetroot	Large serving, 110g (3¾oz)
Cornmeal	Medium serving, 115g (4oz)
Pearl barley	Small serving, 95g (3¼oz)
Wholemeal pasta	½ serving, 85g (3oz) cooked weight
White pasta	⅓ serving, 65g (2¼oz) cooked weight
Brown rice	Small serving, 70g (2½oz) cooked weight
White rice	⅓ serving, 45g (1½oz) cooked weight
Couscous	⅓ serving, 45g (1½oz) soaked weight

Food	Serving size
Broad beans	Small serving, 30g (1oz)
Corn on the cob	½ cob, 60g (2oz)
Boiled potato	3 small, 75g (2¾oz)
Baked potato	½, 60g (2oz)
French fries	Tiny portion, 45g (1½oz)
Sweet potato	½, 60g (2oz)

As you can see, there are some high and some low 'value' foods in this list. The stated portions of Kamut bulgur (which takes only eight minutes to cook) and quinoa (which takes fifteen minutes) will certainly fill you up. The former is delicious on its own, whereas the latter ideally needs some sort of flavouring, but it is a very good source of protein. Wholemeal pasta and brown rice are both much better options than the white alternatives. Similarly, swedes, carrots and squashes are all preferable to potatoes. And boiled potato is better than baked potato, which is better than French fries.

Of course, some keto extremists demonise each and every one of these foods. However, a meta-analysis of some thirty trials revealed that people who eat pasta as part of a low GL diet are no more likely to put on weight than those who cut it out entirely. In fact, low GL pasta eaters tend to lose weight as long as they consume no more than three servings a week.[62]

Beans and Lentils

It's telling that many of the world's fattest nations have shunned beans and lentils over the past hundred years or so. They are missing out because these are the best foods for balancing your blood sugar and providing the perfect combination of protein and carbohydrate. It's mostly due to this rare double-whammy that they have such low GL scores, although lentils and soya also contain a substance that prevents the digestion of amylose, which retards its release even further. Moreover, soya may help your arteries by lowering the level of 'bad' LDL cholesterol: just one serving a day, as either soya milk or tofu, can result in a 10 per cent reduction.

The portion sizes of beans and lentils can be quite generous because you are getting both protein and carbohydrate from a single food source. However, if one of these foods is the meal's primary source of protein, combine it with half the usual portion of carb-rich food. For example, if you make a lentil casserole for two people, use one cup of uncooked lentils and only half a cup of uncooked brown rice. Of course, you need to do this because you are getting quite a lot of carbs – as well as protein – from the lentils.

All the portions in the table below provide the full 7 GL allowance for the carb-rich sector of the plate, so you will need to reduce the quantity if you have some starchy vegetables, too. (A can contains 225–245g (8–8½oz) of beans, and 200g (7oz) of canned beans is roughly equivalent to 40g (1½oz) of dried beans.)

Food	Serving size
Soya beans	4 cans
Pinto/borlotti beans	1 can
Lentils	¾ can
Baked beans	¾ can
Butter beans	¾ can
Split peas	¾ can
Kidney beans	⅔ can
Chickpeas	½ can

If you are not vegetarian, you may be quite unfamiliar with beans and lentils. Although most people have encountered dhal, baked beans, hummus and/or cassoulet, many have never thrown a packet or a tin of lentils or beans into their shopping basket. But these are immensely satisfying, flavourful foods that feature prominently in all of the world's great cuisines. They are also the main ingredients in countless mouth-watering dishes in the Hybrid Diet, from Trout with Puy Lentils and Roasted Tomatoes on the Vine (page 350) to Borlotti Bolognese (page 344) and Chickpea and Spinach Curry (page 347).

Non-starchy vegetables

Now it is time to move on to the other half of the lunch/dinner plate, where we find the 'unlimited vegetables'. Of course, there are *some* limits, but even a generous portion of any of these foods will amount to less than 2 GL. For instance, you could have a whole cupful of peas as part of your meal.

We have listed some of the vast range of options below, with the best all-rounders in bold. (See page 197 for those that also pack the biggest polyphenol/antioxidant/sirtuin activator punch.)

- Artichokes
- **Asparagus**
- Aubergine
- **Avocado**
- Beansprouts
- **Broccoli**
- Brussels sprouts
- **Cabbage**
- Cauliflower
- Celery
- Courgette
- Cucumber
- Endive
- Fennel
- Garlic
- Green beans
- **Kale**
- Lettuce
- Mangetout
- Mushrooms
- **Onion**
- Peas
- Peppers
- Radish
- Runner beans
- Rocket
- Spinach
- Spring onions
- Tomato
- Watercress

To recap, in general, aim to eat two servings of non-starchy vegetables (half a plate), one serving of starchy vegetables and one serving of protein-rich food for both lunch and dinner. If you stick to these proportions, you will feel full at the end of every meal and may well make it all the way through to the next one without ever feeling hungry. And if hunger does strike, you can always treat yourself to a healthy snack.

Top Tips to Lower Your Daily GL

- Add lemon juice to meals

- Liquidise solid food to make soup, as this is more filling

- Soak oats or eat them as porridge

- Chew each mouthful at least twenty times and sip water throughout the meal

- Put your fork down on the plate between mouthfuls

- Add a spoonful of oat bran

- Never add sweet sauces

- Wait thirty minutes before eating something sweet

- Save your dessert until it's time for a snack and include some protein

The Vegetarian Option

If you are a strict vegetarian, you will need to eat more beans, lentils, soya products (such as tofu and tempeh) and Quorn than either meat eaters or pescatarians to achieve the Hybrid Diet's protein intake target (see Chapter 24 for more details). A serving size of tofu for a main meal is 160g (5¾oz) – roughly three-quarters of a packet. Many of the chicken and fish recipes in Part 5 can be adapted by using tofu or tofu steak instead, and a number of recipes feature beans and lentils.

Fats and oils

The slow carb phase is not low fat, so you'll be able to eat enough to keep you satisfied. But it is important to use the right fats in the right ways.

- If you want to make a savoury dish creamier, try adding a teaspoon of tahini or a tablespoon of coconut milk or coconut cream.

- Use either a good quality olive oil or walnut oil, which is high in omega-3, for salad dressings. These oils need to be cold pressed and stored in a light-proof container, ideally in the fridge. Some brands make a health claim on the label regarding the protection of blood lipids from oxidative stress. Treat this as a guarantee of quality, because these oils must have a polyphenol content (hydroxytyrosol) in excess of 250mg per kg of oil. You can lightly drizzle these oils directly onto vegetables in place of butter.

- Use a small amount of butter, ghee, coconut butter or olive oil for steam frying and sautéing. Coconut butter adds great flavour to steam fries.

Cooking Methods

Cooking time and temperature increase a food's glycemic load because they both speed up the release of sugar. Therefore, we recommend eating food that is as close to raw as possible. When you do cook, try to use 'wet' cooking methods (such as steaming) rather than 'dry' (such as baking), as these have less impact on GL.[63]

Don't worry – following these principles doesn't condemn you to endless salads. You can steam, steam fry, boil and poach many foods without cooking them to death. You can even bake, grill, sauté and stir fry, on occasion, but try to avoid frying and especially deep frying.

Steaming

This is the best way to cook leafy, green, non-starchy vegetables, because it preserves a lot of their vitamins and minimises GL increase. Steaming is also great for fish, although you will probably want to use another method for starchy vegetables, which require longer cooking, and red meat. Many different kinds of steamers are available, or you can improvise with a colander, pot and lid.

Boiling

This raises the GL more than steaming, but less than baking. The impact can be kept to a minimum by using as little water as possible, keeping the lid on, and cooking the food as whole as possible. Also, eat your vegetables *al dente* – a little crisp, not soft.

Steam frying

The main advantages of steam frying are that more of the nutrients are preserved because the cooking temperature is so much lower than frying, and you use a fraction of the oil (or none at all). It also enhances the food's flavour. As with boiling and regular steaming, aim to keep vegetables *al dente*.

Use either a shallow pan or a deep frying pan with a thick base and a lid that seals well. If you want to steam fry without any oil, first add two tablespoons of liquid – water, vegetable stock, soy sauce and/or some of the sauce you are using for the dish – to the pan. Add some vegetables as soon as the liquid comes to the boil, sauté rapidly for a minute or two, turn the heat up, add one or two more tablespoons of the liquid, then fit the lid. Add the remaining ingredients after one minute, then turn the heat down after a couple of minutes and continue to steam until fully cooked.

Alternatively, you can add anything between a teaspoon and a tablespoon of olive oil, butter or coconut oil to the pan, warm it, add the ingredients and sauté. After a couple of minutes, add two tablespoons of liquid (as above) and clamp on the lid. Steam until fully cooked.

Poaching

This is similar to steam frying without the sautéing. We recommend using water-based sauces to give your meals a big boost of flavour: for example, try cooking fish in vegetable broth flavoured with ginger, garlic, lemongrass, spices and wine (the alcohol boils off).

Waterless Cooking

This requires specially designed pans in which you 'boil' foods by steaming them in their own juices and 'fry' foods with no oil. Both methods are excellent ways to preserve both nutrients and flavour.

Baking

Despite its drawbacks (see above), baking can be useful if the food is large and has a thick skin (such as a whole pumpkin).

Avoid coating the food with oil, because this will oxidise during cooking, which creates free radicals (highly reactive, harmful molecules). You can roast a potato without the addition of any oil. Remember, the higher the temperature and the longer cooking time, the higher the GL becomes.

Frying

All frying should be kept to a minimum, and avoid deep frying altogether. Use butter or coconut oil (saturated fat) or olive oil (mono-unsaturated fat), rather than other vegetable oils (poly-unsaturated fat), because the latter are much more prone to oxidation.

Grilling

Using this method for foods that contain fat is less harmful than frying, but charring will still create free radicals. Therefore, try to avoid barbecued and especially burned food.

Microwaving

Although microwaving is fast, and the food cooks in its own water, which means that more of the water-soluble vitamins B and C are preserved, there are some significant drawbacks to this method of cooking. Fat particles reach very high temperatures, so avoid microwaving oily fish as all of the essential fats it contains will be destroyed. And remember that microwaves emit electromagnetic radiation to a distance of several metres. It is advisable to use lower voltage and heat settings coupled with longer cooking times, and cover dishes to encourage steaming (although you must leave gaps for some steam to escape).

Top Tips for Healthy Cooking

- Ensure that all of your food is as fresh and unprocessed as possible.

- Eat more raw food: be adventurous, for instance by trying raw beetroot and carrot tops in salads.

- Cook foods in their natural, whole state, then slice or blend before serving.

- Use as little water as possible during cooking, preferably during steaming, poaching or steam frying.

- Minimise fried food in your diet.

- Favour slower, low temperature cooking methods.

- Never eat overcooked, charred or burned food.

Desserts

We recommend avoiding all desserts, sweets and sweetened drinks (including fruit juice) in the first two weeks of the slow carb phase if your aim is to take control of your blood sugar balance. Once this has stabilised, you can allow yourself a daily allowance of 5 GLs for drinks and desserts. This means that you should still avoid desserts when eating out, because almost all restaurant sweets and puddings are loaded with white sugar and processed fat.

If you are used to eating a lot of desserts, or if you are insulin resistant, you will probably crave something sweet at the end of every meal, but it is crucial to break this habit if you want to stop your blood sugar seesawing. Fortunately, most people find that the cravings disappear after just three days. To stop them returning, it's a good idea to limit desserts to just one a week (perhaps as a treat at the weekend) after your initial sugar-free fortnight. Alternatively, continue to avoid them altogether and eat a low GL bar, such as Fruitus Oat & Mixed Berry (roughly 5 GLs), instead.

When to Eat

As we mentioned at the beginning of this chapter, breakfast is the most important meal of the day, and you must ensure that it contains the requisite amount of protein. Eggs are an easy way to achieve this, but if you prefer cereal, you can always add ground seeds and milk (or almond milk). This sort of breakfast will stop you experiencing hunger pangs later in the day.

In the evening, aim to finish dinner at least two hours before you go to bed. Of course, you must also ensure that this final meal of the day is low GL, with sufficient protein. Including beans, lentils or chickpeas as your 7 GL carb portion will help to keep your blood sugar balanced throughout the night and will even lower the GL of your breakfast the next day.

Don't eat anything after dinner and aim for a minimum of eleven hours between dinner and breakfast. You can extend this to thirteen or even fifteen hours if you find this comfortable (see Chapter 15). Ensure that you get a good night's sleep because research has shown that insufficient sleep disrupts the body's appetite hormones.[64]

Sample Menus

We have devised five days of menus to help you get started in the slow carb phase. We give the GL of each dish plus the daily total, up to a maximum of 40 GLs a day. This means you have an extra 5 GLs for a drink each day. See Chapter 29 for drink recommendations. As for desserts, as mentioned above, avoid these for at least the first two weeks. Thereafter, you'll find some excellent low GL ideas in Patrick's *Low GL Diet Cookbook* or *Ten Secrets of 100% Health Cookbook*.

All the dishes in capitals can be found in Part 5.

Day 1

Breakfast	Get Up & Go with CarboSlow, with milk or low carb almond milk and berries **8 GL**
Snack	A piece of fruit, plus five almonds or a dessertspoon of pumpkin seeds **5 GL**
Lunch	Chestnut and Butter Bean Soup **4 GL**
Snack	A small, no-added-sugar, plain yoghurt (150g), plus berries or soya berry yoghurt **3.5 GL**
Dinner	Thai Lamb Red Curry **8 GL**
	Total: 28.5 GL

Day 2

Breakfast	Oat and chia porridge **10 GL**
Snack	A small serving of yesterday's Chestnut and Butter Bean Soup **4 GL**
Lunch	Walnut and Three Bean Salad **3 GL**
Snack	A slice of Apple and Almond Cake **5 GL**
Dinner	Trout with Puy Lentils and Roasted Tomatoes on the Vine **10 GL**
	Total: 32 GL

Day 3

Breakfast	Yoghurt and berries with chopped almonds **5 GL**
Snack	A thin slice of bread or two oatcakes and a quarter of a small tub of hummus (50g) **5 GL**

Lunch	Apple and Tuna Salad **4 GL**
Snack	A slice of Low GL Carrot and Walnut Cake **5 GL**
Dinner	Sticky Mustard Salmon Fillets **10 GL**
	Total: 29 GL

Day 4

Breakfast	Scrambled eggs on oatcakes or pumpernickel bread **9 GL**
Snack	Crudités (sliced carrot, pepper, cucumber or celery) and hummus **5 GL**
Lunch	Summer Pea and Mint Soup **3 GL**
Snack	A piece of fruit, plus five almonds or a dessertspoon of pumpkin seeds **5 GL**
Dinner	Kamut Spaghetti with Chestnut Mushrooms and Truffle Oil **10 GL**
	Total: 32 GL

Day 5

Breakfast	Low GL Granola **5 GL**
Snack	A thin slice of rye bread or two oatcakes, plus sugar-free peanut butter **5 GL**
Lunch	Quinoa Tabbouleh **8 GL**
Snack	A slice of Apple and Almond Cake **5 GL**
Dinner	Garlic Chilli Prawns with Pak Choi **10 GL**
	Total: 33 GL

Chapter 24

Going Hybrid for Vegetarians, Vegans and Pescatarians

The slow carb phase of the Hybrid Diet is easy to follow if you don't eat meat or dairy products. The high fat phase can be a bit more tricky for vegans, but it is still feasible. Meanwhile, pescatarians will find both phases no trouble at all.

At the time of writing, there were an estimated 3.5 million vegans in the UK, about an equal number of vegetarians, and possibly even more pescatarians, and the figures were growing for all three. Therefore, we can say that at least 10 per cent of the UK population have turned away from meat for one reason or another. Other developed countries, most notably the United States, have similar proportions of non-meat eaters. Many have been motivated to make the switch by the profiteering and lack of compassion of the meat industry and/or the obvious health benefits of going vegetarian.

Those health benefits certainly look impressive. One recent

review of all the available evidence concluded that vegetarians are 33–50 per cent less likely than non-vegetarians to develop diabetes, while people in the top fifth for animal protein intake increase their risk by 13 per cent.[65] According to the researchers, 'substituting 5% of energy intake from vegetable protein for animal protein was associated with a 23% reduced risk of diabetes'. Other studies have shown that eating a healthy, plant-based diet also lowers cholesterol, blood pressure, insulin and HbA1c levels, and inflammation.[66] What's not to like?

Well, there are risks, especially for those who adopt one of the more extreme vegan diets: lack of vitamins B_{12} and D, zinc and omega-3s are all high on the list of potential issues. This can be especially problematic during pregnancy, as the developing foetus needs sufficient quantities of all these nutrients. Vegetarian women tend to have less than optimal levels of zinc,[67] while vegans can be deficient in vitamins D and B_{12}.[68] Both groups' omega-3 levels are often less than ideal, too.[69]

Can Vegans Get Enough Omega-3?

On average, vegetarians have 60 per cent less omega-3 than people who eat fish, and even lower levels of brain-friendly DHA – the most important omega-3 fat – which is found in abundance in seafood. The general view is that only between 5 and 10 per cent of alpha linolenic acid (ALA) – the vegetarian form of omega-3 that is found in the likes of chia and flax seeds – is converted into EPA, and even less is converted into DHA (see illustration overleaf). From these we make anti-inflammatory prostaglandins. DHA is also structural, used to build the brain.

The omega-3 fats

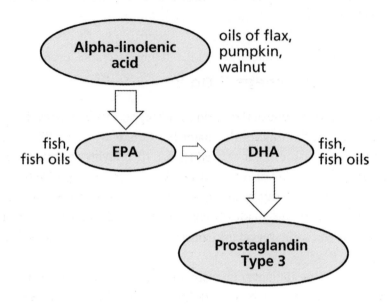

In 2010, the University of East Anglia monitored the omega-3 intake of more than 14,000 people in Norfolk.[70] The same team also analysed blood plasma levels of the more potent long-chain fats (EPA, DPA and DHA) in a third of the participants to determine the quantities that actually enter the bloodstream from the diet. One of their conclusions was that dark green, leafy vegetables provide significant amounts of omega-3, as does meat, but both trail far behind oily fish. Unsurprisingly, then, as consumption of fish – and especially oily fish – increases, so do blood plasma levels of EPA and DHA. (Supplement takers can achieve very high levels, too.)

Interestingly, though, the difference in levels between vegetarians and pescatarians – and especially between female vegetarians and pescatarians – was not nearly as great as might have been expected. The inference is that the body must produce more EPA and DHA from vegetable sources of ALA when it is deprived of direct sources of these fats. And it is possible that women are better at this task because of their higher oestrogen levels. This makes evolutionary sense, as EPA and DHA are so vital during pregnancy.

How Much Omega-3 Do You Need?

Joseph Hibbeln, one of the world's leading experts on omega-3 and disease risk, has stated: 'The majority of the population (98–99%) are protected from ... increased risk of chronic illnesses [with an intake of] 2g a day of EPA and DHA.' A 100g serving of salmon provides roughly this amount. A daily omega-3 supplement provides about 700mg, so ideally combine this with three servings of oily fish and some vegetarian sources of ALA (such as chia or flax seeds) each week.

There are some natural vegan sources of DHA, derived from seaweed and algae, which work just as well,[71] but the amount of DHA is less than fish oils, and they provide little EPA. We recommend vegans do take omega-3 supplements.

On the other hand, even if your diet includes a large amount of omega-3, you may be getting *too much* omega-6, which is found in high concentrations in hot climate seeds, such as sesame and sunflower. Your brain functions best on a two to one ratio of omega-6 to omega-3. Most Western diets are closer to fifteen to one! So, rather than using sunflower or sesame seeds and oil, switch to walnut, chia or flax oil for salad dressings, olive oil for cooking, and ground chia, flax or pumpkin seeds on cereals and in smoothies.

Problems with Protein

In Chapter 21 we explained the dangers of getting too much protein in the form of meat. Conversely, it can be difficult for vegans to get *enough* protein in their diet. By contrast, pescatarians have the best of both worlds: none of the health dangers of eating modern, processed meat products as well as easy access to essential fats and protein.

Vegans in the Slow Carb Phase

Nevertheless, we appreciate that some readers will not want to include any animal products, including fish, in the Hybrid Diet. As we mentioned at the start of this chapter, this is less straightforward than the pescatarian approach, but it can be done.

In the slow carb phase, choose a good vegetarian source of protein for that quarter of the plate. However, as all vegetarian proteins contain at least some carbohydrate, you will need to increase the protein portion and make a corresponding reduction to the carb-rich sector. Use the illustration as a rough guide.

The vegan food plate

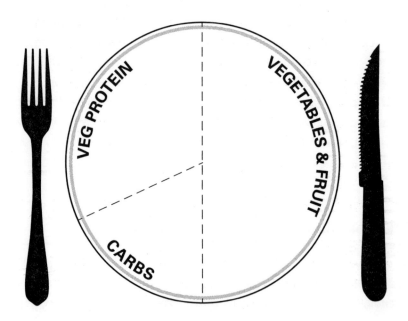

For instance, if you have a 5 GL portion of beans as your source of protein, you might need to halve the standard serving of starchy vegetables. However, some beans contain more protein (and therefore fewer carbs) than others, so you will need to factor this into your calculations.

In the table below you can see how much of various beans you need to eat, both to achieve 15 grams of protein, the ideal amount for a meal, and to provide 7 GL of carbs, which is the amount to aim for in the slow carb phase. However, in the high fat phase you only have an allowance of 15 GLs, or 5 GLs per meal. This is not an issue if you choose beans at the top half of the chart below. For example, half a can of lentils would be about 5 GLs and give you almost enough protein. Soya beans and soya-based foods, such as tofu, are also a great choice in the high fat phase, Peas, pinto beans, borlotti beans, lentils and butter beans are all good alternatives, whereas haricot and black-eyed beans should be avoided, or very much limited in the slow carb phase. Less than a quarter of a can of black-eyed beans is already 7 GLs.

Food	Serving size for 15g protein	Serving size for 7 GLs
Soya beans	⅕ can (40g)	4 cans (1050g)
Peas	¼ can (300g)	2 cans (525g)
Pinto beans	¼ can (70g)	1 can (262g)
Borlotti beans	¼ can (65g)	1 can (262g)
Lentils	⅔ (170g)	¾ can (210g)
Butter beans	⅔ can (190g)	¾ can (175g)
Split peas	¼ can (60g)	¾ can (175g)
Baked beans	1⅓ cans (310g)	⅔ can (150g)
Kidney beans	¾ can(175g)	⅔ can (150g)
Chickpeas	⅓ can (80g)	½ can (132g)
Flageolet beans	¾ can (210g)	½ can (116g)
Haricot beans	1 can (250g)	⅓ can (87g)
Black-eyed beans	½ can (165g)	⅓ can (87g)

(A 400g can provides approx. 240g of beans)

Chestnut and Butter Bean Soup is flavourful, totally vegan, can be made in five minutes and is only 4 GLs per serving. Other excellent vegan protein options are Quorn, soya mince and tofu. The latter, which is available in several delicious forms (try marinated tofu), can be substituted for fish or chicken in many of the recipes in Part 5, or try our Spicy Pumpkin and Tofu Soup. Our recommended tofu serving size for a main meal is 160g (5¾oz) – roughly three-quarters of a packet.

Pescatarians, Vegans and Vegetarians in the High Fat Phase

It is quite simple to achieve ketosis by eating oily fish, avocados, coconut oil and high quality, polyphenol-rich olive oil, plus the right nuts and seeds (pecan, Brazil, macadamia, walnut and chia are best). If you include plenty of these in your diet, there's no need to go anywhere near red meat or dairy products.

In truth, it is very hard to go keto on a completely vegan diet. Without oily fish, eggs or dairy products as sources of fat and protein you must rely on beans, lentils, nuts and seeds for protein and you'll need to eat lots of avocados – probably two or more a day – and load up on nuts butters, coconut oil and C8 oil, with lots of oily salad dressings, including liberal use of tahini.

Also, minimise your consumption of a few high GL starchy vegetables, such as potatoes, sweet potatoes and parsnips. The best veggies are broccoli, cauliflower, cabbage, Brussels sprouts, kale, asparagus, artichokes, spinach, rocket and watercress, plus runner beans, broad beans and peas, as well as garlic and red onions. Don't go overboard on carrots, and certainly not carrot juice.

Any more than 50g of carbs per day will interfere with ketosis, so stay below that line and you'll have plenty of room for the higher vegetable protein, lower carb foods such as tofu, tempeh and quinoa, and you'll still be able to eat the occasional handful of blueberries and blackberries.

Eat More

- Fish* (sardines, non-farmed salmon, mackerel, herring, Arctic cod, halibut)
- Organic, free range eggs*
- Nuts and seeds (pecan, Brazil, macadamia, chia)
- Nut and seed oils such as tahini and almond butter
- Avocados (one per day)
- Coconut oil
- Ghee (but not after a breast or prostate cancer diagnosis)*
- Cacao butter
- Polyphenol-rich olive oil and olives
- Non-starchy vegetables
- Mushrooms
- Berries (especially blueberries)
- Quinoa, tofu, tempeh and lentils

* Unless vegan.

Eat Less

- Grain

- Sugar (avoid completely, except for xylitol, erythritol or stevia)

- High sugar fruit (bananas, grapes, raisins and dates)

- Dairy (and no 'low fat', non-organic products)

Sample Menus

Below, we list a number of vegetarian, vegan and pescatarian options for all three meals, snacks and desserts. Remember, though, you can also substitute tofu, soya mince or Quorn for many of the fish and chicken recipes in Part 5.

Breakfast

Scrambled eggs made with olive oil, ghee or coconut oil, plus mushrooms or smoked salmon
Scrambled tofu (with a couple of oatcakes if not aiming for rapid ketosis)
Huevos rancheros with avocado and salsa
Chia porridge made with unsweetened soya or almond milk and coconut yoghurt
Get Up & Go, plus berries, coconut oil/cream, chia, cinnamon and cacao butter, diluted with half water, half unsweetened soya or almond milk

Lunch and Dinner

Tofu or tempeh with lots of non-starchy vegetables
Lentil and vegetable hotpot
Chestnut and Butter Bean Soup (page 339)
Soya mince chilli with kidney beans
Wholemeal Kamut Pasta with Borlotti Bolognese (page 344)
Fish with salad or steamed vegetables
Fish, nuts, green salad and avocado
Fish soup

Snacks

Raw nuts and seeds (e.g. pecans, Brazils or pumpkin seeds) with
or without berries
Yoghurt (soya, coconut or organic cow's milk) with seeds
and berries
Avocado with hummus or olive oil
Crudités (celery is best; pepper and carrot in moderation) with
guacamole or taramasalata
(Tip: Jimmy Moore and Maria Emmerich's *The Ketogenic
Cookbook* has dozens of healthy ketogenic recipes, many of which
are vegan or vegetarian.[72])

Chapter 25

Hybrid Support Micronutrients

S o far, our journey into the body's metabolism has focused almost exclusively on macronutrients: that is, the foods that are transformed into either ketones or glucose for fuel. But how does this actually happen, and how can you support your metabolism to turn it into a mean, lean, energy-generating machine?

Every chemical step along the way requires enzymes, which are made within the body and ultimately enable the release of the pure energy that is stored in food. Something is wrong if you are storing that energy as fat, rather than feeling energised.

All of these enzymes depend on keys – known as co-factors – to make them work. The illustration opposite is based on a very similar one in Chapter 13 (see page 121), which illustrated how your body makes ketones and glucose and then turns these fuels into energy (ATP), but this time we have added the micronutrients that lubricate the whole process. The doors of your metabolism won't open properly without these keys, so they are crucial for good health.

Micronutrients that are necessary for efficient metabolism

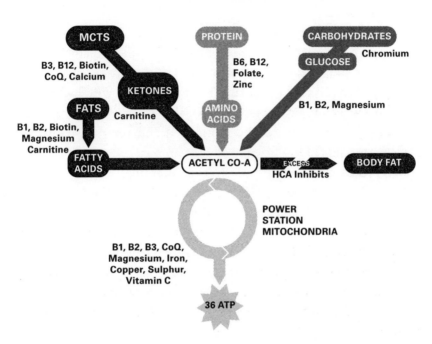

B and C Vitamins: The Energy Nutrients

A quick glance at the illustration above reveals the importance of a lot of B vitamins, vitamin C and a number of minerals. Many people assume that we get all the nutrients we need from a well-balanced diet. But what is 'need'? And what is a 'well-balanced diet'? These vague terms lead to complacency . . . and deficiency.

By contrast, if you ask a more precise question, such as, 'What is the optimal intake of vitamin C for optimal health?' – that is, lots of energy and as little disease as possible – the answer might be anything between 500 and 2,000mg. Even the lower of these two figures is many times higher than the RDA (recommended daily allowance; or, as we term it, ridiculous dietary arbitrary!) of 80mg. The 'average' person gets just 100mg of vitamin C from their food, which means that a significant minority will get far less.

Theoretically, it may seem like a good idea to optimise your body's biochemistry, but what difference will it really make? Well, the simple answer is that you will have more energy – both mental and physical – and burn more fat. People with metabolic syndrome shunt energy-rich glucose into storage as fat, but this unhealthy diversion can be minimised and reversed with the right amounts of 'traffic control' nutrients.

As you can see from the illustration, vitamin C is a co-factor – a key stage in the energy-making process whether the fuel is glucose or ketones. It is also vital for the manufacture of adrenal and thyroid hormones, both of which instruct the cells to make more energy. Unsurprisingly, then, many studies have linked low levels of vitamin C to increased fatigue. For example, researchers at the University of Alabama Medical Center monitored the vitamin C intake of more than 400 volunteers and asked them to rate their 'fatigability'. Those who consumed less than 100mg per day had an average score of 0.81. Conversely, those who consumed more than 400mg a day we half as tired, with an average score of just 0.41.[73] 'Individuals consuming the generally accepted RDA for vitamin C report approximately twice the fatigue symptomatology as those taking about sevenfold the RDA,' concluded the lead researcher, Dr Emanuel Cheraskin.

One of the knock-on effects of metabolic syndrome – which plays such a key role in the undesirable twenty-first-century cocktail of weight gain, diabetes, heart disease and Alzheimer's – is a sluggish thyroid. The thyroid produces thyroxine – a hormone that tells the body's cells to make more energy. If levels of thyroxine start to fall, the brain secretes thyroid stimulating hormone (TSH), which tells the thyroid to buck up! So, high TSH and low thyroxine levels indicate you've got a sluggish thyroid gland (a condition that is known as hypothyroidism). Dr William Jubiz, from Cali, Colombia, suspected that this might be reversed by supplementing vitamin C, so he gave thirty-one of his hypothyroid patients an extra 500mg for three months. TSH levels improved in all but one of the participants in the trial, and returned to normal in seventeen of them.[74]

B vitamins also play vital roles in the energy-making process. However, many people are deficient in at least some of them – most notably vitamin B_{12} and biotin – especially as they get older. One UK study found that 40 per cent of people over the age of sixty-one have insufficient B_{12},[75] while a recent Irish study reported that one in eight are deficient and only 3 per cent of those aged over fifty have optimal levels.[76] In part, this may be due to the fact that metformin, the most commonly prescribed diabetes drug, makes B_{12} harder to absorb. Proton pump inhibitors, such as omeprazole, which the NHS prescribes for millions of people with stomach acid issues at an annual cost of more than £100 million (over £2 billion globally), are even worse in this respect.[77] In addition to affecting the body's absorption of B_{12} and therefore reducing your energy levels, some studies have suggested that these drugs shorten life expectancy.[78] If you are a poor absorber of B_{12} – which is only found in animal products, such as meat, fish, eggs and dairy – you will need to supplement literally hundreds of times more than the RDA of 2mcg. When researchers tested how much supplemental B_{12} was needed to correct even mild deficiency, the answer was more than 500mcg a day![79] It is impossible to eat this amount, so supplementing (or injections) is the only option.

Another crucial B vitamin is niacin (B_3), which is converted into nicotinamide adenine dinucleotide (NAD) – a compound that is responsible for transporting the packets of energy in our food into our cells' mitochondria. NAD levels decline as we age, but tend to increase when the body is in ketosis, because we need more. Such increases help the body to repair itself during autophagy and improve insulin function. Supplementing niacin helps to optimise NAD levels because we need at least 50mg a day (almost three times the RDA).

Another important B vitamin – biotin – is often neglected because it can be synthesized in the gut if the right bacteria are present. However, you must ensure that you have sufficient quantities because it is an absolutely vital component in the metabolism of ketones. In addition, deficiency results in damage to mitochondria and DNA as well as accelerated ageing, and you can't make red blood cells without it. Yet, biotin deficiency is remarkably common: one study estimated that 40 per cent of pregnant women who do not take a multivitamin have insufficient levels.[80] Ensure that your multivitamin provides at least 50mcg. Some 'high potency' supplements include biotin and another important nutrient – folate – along with B_1, B_2, B_3, B_6, and B_{12}.

Supplementing vitamin C and these B vitamins can make a significant difference to how you feel and your energy levels. One 2011 trial gave a group of volunteers either a multivitamin or a placebo. After twenty-eight days, those taking the supplement exhibited greater physical and mental stamina, better concentration and more alertness than those taking the placebo.[81]

Co-enzyme Q

Co-enzyme Q (Co-Q) is a crucial ingredient in the final stage of the body's energy-making process – the electron transport system – because it controls the flow of oxygen, making the whole procedure more efficient. In addition, it boosts the enzyme HMG CoA synthase, which plays a pivotal role in the metabolism of ketones. By contrast, statins suppress this enzyme, which is why their side effects often include muscle pain and fatigue. In one trial, fifty patients who had been taking statins for two years were taken off the medication after complaining of muscle pain. Their symptoms improved dramatically when they were given Co-Q.[82]

Co-Q also mops up free radicals, which accelerate the ageing process and damage artery walls, among other harmful effects, if left unattended. These dangerous compounds are created during normal metabolism but also when we come into contact with pollution, the sun's radiation, cigarette smoke and charred, fried food.

There is no evidence that supplementing Co-Q has any adverse effects (even when it is taken in very high quantities over a long period of time), while the benefits may be profound. In one study, volunteers who were given 300mg of Co-Q for eight days reported greater energy and demonstrated improved performance during twice-daily, intensive, two-hour physical workouts.[83] Many other studies have shown that Co-Q has a positive impact on heart and artery health.[84] Therefore, we recommend ongoing supplementation of 30–60mg of Co-Q each day, or 90–120mg if you are taking statins or have been diagnosed with cardiovascular disease. Many different products are available, but we recommend those that are oil soluble, as these are most readily absorbed by the body.

A number of foods contain Co-Q, but not always in the form that our bodies can use. There are ten different types – from $Co-Q_1$ to $Co-Q_{10}$. Yeast, for example, contains $Co-Q_6$ and $Co-Q_7$. However, only $Co-Q_{10}$ is found in human tissues, so this is the form that you should supplement. The 'lower' forms of Co-Q should not be neglected, because the liver can convert them into $Co-Q_{10}$, although we seem to lose this ability as we age, which is why supplementation is so important for elderly people.

The best dietary sources of $Co-Q_{10}$ are meat, fish (especially sardines), eggs, spinach, broccoli, alfalfa, potato, soya beans and oil, wheat (especially wheatgerm), rice bran, buckwheat, millet and most beans, nuts and seeds. The table overleaf gives the amounts of $Co-Q_{10}$ in a variety of foods.

The Best Sources of Co-Q$_{10}$

Food	Amount (mg per g)	Food	Amount (mg per g)
Meat		**Beans**	
Beef	.031	Green beans	.0058
Pork	.024–.041	Soya beans	.0029
Chicken	.021	Aduki beans	.0022
		Soya oil	.092
Fish			
Sardines.	064	**Nuts and seeds**	
Mackerel	.043	Peanuts	.027
Flat fish	.005	Sesame seeds	.023
		Walnuts	.019
Grains			
Wheatgerm	.0035	**Vegetables**	
Millet	.0015	Spinach	.010
Buckwheat	.0013	Broccoli	.008
Rice bran	.0054	Peppers	.003
		Carrots	.002

Carnitine: Essential in the High Fat Phase

Like Co-Q$_{10}$, carnitine is known as a 'semi-essential' nutrient, which means that your body can make it, but it cannot make enough for optimal health, especially if you are getting on in years. In addition, though, you need more carnitine when you are in ketosis because it plays a key role in both burning fat for energy and feeding fat into the body's ketogenic furnaces. Therefore, carnitine deficiency is quite common among people on a ketogenic diet. For instance, a study of children with epilepsy who had been following a strict high fat diet found that 17 per cent were carnitine deficient.[85]

Similarly, deficiency can become a problem when people burn more calories than they eat, even over a relatively short period of time. One study analysed the carnitine levels in a group of soldiers who skied fifty-one kilometres in four days – an extreme test of physical endurance in which the participants burned more than double the calories they were able to consume. The more energy they expended, the more carnitine they needed to transport fatty acids into their cells' mitochondria for fuel.[86]

Even when the body is not in ketosis, more than half of the heart's energy needs are met by burning fat; and, since it has to work hard every second of every day, it demands a steady, constant supply. Carnitine is the delivery boy that carries the fatty acids this vital organ needs. It also removes the toxic by-products that are created when the fuel is burned.

A number of trials show that carnitine supplementation can increase ketone levels and promote weight loss.[87]

We recommend taking carnitine at least twice a day, because it remains in the body for no more than a few hours. If you want to accelerate your entry into ketosis, we suggest a total of 250–500mg per day. If you are burning ketones – for example, if you are an endurance athlete – take at least 500mg per day, divided into two or more doses. However, you could easily double this, as there no toxicity concerns with supplementing up to 2,000mg a day (which is probably the maximum you would ever need in the high fat phase). Some supplements provide Co-Q$_{10}$ with carnitine (see Resources).

Carnitine is especially helpful if you drink alcohol, have chronic fatigue, engage in endurance sports or suffer from low libido. So, it's good for your heart, good for your brain, good on the track or ski runs and good for your love life ... especially if you plan to be in ketosis for an extended period of time.

Hydroxycitric Acid: The Thai Secret

Thailand, and South-East Asia in general, has some of the lowest rates of obesity, diabetes, cancer and heart disease in the world. In part, this may be due to the prevalence of tamarind fruit in the traditional Thai diet.

There is a compound called hydroxycitric acid (HCA) in the rind of the tamarind that suppresses the key enzyme in the body's fat storage process (ATP-citrate lyase). This has a significant positive impact on levels of 'bad' LDL cholesterol in the blood, fatty liver and inflammation, risk of heart disease and blood sugar issues associated with diabetes.[88] It also cranks up activity in the thyroid, which prompts an increase in metabolism, so more fat is burned for energy.[89] In one study, rats that were fed HCA lost significant amounts of weight, experienced better blood sugar control and suffered less inflammation.[90] It also reduces appetite, possibly by boosting the secretion of serotonin.

Moreover, Thomas Seyfried, who has pioneered the use of ketogenic diets in the treatment of brain cancer, believes that HCA may prove to be an important ally in the ongoing battle against glioblastoma. He has reported particularly impressive results when it is combined with alpha-lipoic acid.[91]

We recommend supplementing above 2g of HCA per day (e.g. three doses of 750mg) to aid weight loss. A meta-analysis of nine studies of HCA supplementation reported average weight loss of about 1.2kg (2.7lb) in eight weeks,[92] but participants in trials that gave more than 2g a day fared much better, averaging about 3.5kg over the trial period (roughly 1lb per week). As an example, one team of researchers placed sixty volunteers on a 2,000 calorie diet plus a thirty-minute walking exercise programme and gave them either a placebo or 2,800mg of HCA per day in three equal doses. After eight weeks, those taking HCA had lost 5.4 per cent more body weight and their BMI was 5.2 per cent lower than the placebo group. In addition, their food intake, total cholesterol, LDL cholesterol, triglycerides and serum leptin levels (the hormone that triggers eating) were all significantly lower, while their 'good' HDL cholesterol, serotonin levels and excretion of urinary fat metabolites (a biomarker of fat oxidation) were all significantly higher. No adverse effects were reported.[93] There have been some reports of liver toxicity in other studies, but only among people with diabetes or fatty liver disease, those on potentially liver-toxic medication and/or those who were following extremely low calorie diets. There is no evidence that supplementing HCA causes any harm to people who are in generally good health. Indeed, a major review deemed it safe to use up to 2,800mg a day,[94] which, as we have seen, is enough to support weight loss. Even so, we would err on the side of caution if you have any sort of liver dysfunction or non-alcoholic fatty liver disease.

Elemental Energy

The minerals calcium, magnesium, iron, chromium, zinc and copper are also vital for energy production. The first two are perhaps the most important because all of the body's muscle cells need an adequate supply of both in order to contract and relax efficiently. Fortunately, most Westerners get more than enough calcium in their diet. However, magnesium deficiency is very common among people who eat insufficient quantities of fruit and vegetables.

Three-quarters of the body's enzymes need magnesium. It plays a key role in the Krebs energy-making cycle, is vital for carbohydrate metabolism and helps nerve cells transmit their messages. Symptoms of deficiency include cramp, muscle weakness or tremors, insomnia, nervousness, hyperactivity, depression, confusion, irregular heartbeat, constipation and lack of appetite. The average daily intake in the UK is about 272mg, but we need about 450mg for optimal health. If you are conscientious about eating your greens, and have some nuts and seeds each day, you will probably get about 350mg. Pumpkin seeds are a great source, as are almonds and chia and flax seeds: a small handful provides about 75mg. Nevertheless, it is a good idea to take a daily multivitamin and mineral that gives you at least 100mg of magnesium (plus double that amount of calcium.

Your body needs zinc, together with vitamin B_6, to make the enzymes that digest food.[95] These micronutrients are also essential for the production of insulin. A lack of zinc can disrupt appetite control and even diminish the senses of taste and smell, which can result in a preference for meat, cheese and other foods with strong flavours. Zinc is found in nuts and seeds, meat, fish, eggs, beans and lentils. In addition, these foods are good sources of iron, copper and sulphur, which are also key players in the electron transport system. We recommend supplementing 10mg of zinc, 10mg iron and 0.5mg of copper each day. Onions, garlic and eggs all contain plenty of sulphur, so there is no need to supplement it if you eat these foods.

Chromium Reverses Insulin Resistance

The older you are, the less likely you are to be eating enough chromium.[96] It is an essential mineral that helps stabilise blood sugar by making you more sensitive to insulin,[97] thus reversing insulin resistance. Presumably as a consequence, supplementing chromium has been shown to reduce appetite and promote weight loss,[98] mitigate mood dips[99] and depression,[100] and reduce fatigue in diabetics.[101]

The average daily intake of chromium is less than 50mcg, whereas optimal intake, certainly for those with blood sugar problems, is closer to 200mcg. Diabetics need considerably more – about 600mcg – to resensitise their insulin receptors. It has many other benefits, too. A recent study gave a group of volunteers either 600mcg of chromium or a placebo for four months. At the end of the trial, the chromium group had lower blood glucose both before and after meals; their levels of HbA1c (the key long-term blood sugar marker) and cholesterol were both significantly lower, too.[102] A meta-analysis of twenty-two previous trials reported similar findings.[103]

There are two words of caution, however. First, because chromium often boosts energy, it can make sleep difficult if taken in the evening. Therefore, we recommend one tablet with breakfast, one with lunch and one in the afternoon, before 5 p.m. Second, diabetics often find that their blood sugar has stabilised after taking 600mcg of chromium for a few months. At that point, if your blood sugar becomes too low reduce the dose to around 200mcg.

Chromium is found in relatively high concentrations in whole grains, beans, nuts and seeds, and especially asparagus and mushrooms. (By contrast, 98 per cent of the chromium is removed from white flour in the refining process – another good reason to steer clear of refined foods.) However, you are unlikely to achieve optimal intake from diet alone. Therefore, we recommend supplementation, even if you are not diabetic. Chromium polynicotinate is probably the best form to try, as it also contains niacin (vitamin B_3). The liver uses these two micronutrients to make a substance called glucose tolerance factor, which, as the name suggests, enhances the body's ability to deal with glucose by binding to insulin and increasing its efficiency.[104]

Supplements for Energy

Given that all of these vitamins and minerals boost the body's energy-making processes and therefore reduce the storage of fat, it is logical to assume that guaranteeing optimal daily amounts through supplementation will aid weight loss. But is this the case?

Well, one study monitored three groups of people, all of whom followed a strict low GL diet: those who took no supplements; those who took a basic multivitamin and mineral, plus vitamin C and essential fats; and those who took these plus at least two of chromium, HCA and 5-HTP (the latter boosts serotonin, which controls appetite). Those on the diet alone lost an average of 550g (1¼lb) per week; those who took the basic supplements lost 680g (1½lb) per week; whereas those who took these and the additional supplements lost almost 1kg (2lb) per week.[105]

Ensuring an optimal intake of all the nutrients that play a role in turning food into energy is a key part of the energy equation. Therefore, it can accelerate weight loss and reverse metabolic syndrome and related diseases, such as diabetes. Of course, eating the right kind of food is essential, but supplementation is the best way to guarantee that you will achieve these optimal levels every day.

Top Vitamin and Mineral Tips

- Include foods that are rich in B vitamins (fish, green vegetables, beans, lentils, whole grains, mushrooms, eggs) and vitamin C (green vegetables, berries, citrus fruit) in your diet.

- Eat more good sources of the enzyme $Co-Q_{10}$ (sardines, mackerel, sesame seeds, peanuts, walnuts, beef, pork, chicken, spinach).

- Ensure you get plenty of magnesium (from almonds, chia and pumpkin seeds, green vegetables), calcium (from cheese, almonds, green vegetables, seeds), zinc (from oysters, lamb, nuts, fish, egg yolk, whole grains, almonds, chia seeds) and chromium (from whole grains, beans, nuts, seeds, asparagus, mushrooms).

- Supplement a high potency multivitamin and mineral twice a day to guarantee you get all the B vitamins, magnesium (at least 100mg), zinc (at least 10mg), copper (at least 0.5mg) and iron (at least 10mg) that you need.

- Supplement 500mg to 1g of vitamin C twice a day (no multivitamin contains this much, which is why you have to take it separately).

- Consider supplementing Co-Q_{10} and certainly supplement carnitine, especially if you are over fifty, taking statins, following a ketogenic diet and/or dealing with any of the following: cardiovascular disease, cancer or cognitive decline. Aim for 30–120mg of Co-Q_{10} and 250mg–2g of carnitine, depending on your condition. Some supplements combine these (see Resources).

- Consider supplementing chromium for better blood sugar and appetite control, and carnitine and HCA to aid weight loss. You will need 200mcg of chromium up to three times a day if you are diabetic, and 750mg of HCA up to three times a day for weight loss. Some supplements combine these (see Resources).

Chapter 26

Biohacking Your Ketone/ Glucose Balance

S hedding pounds and enjoying extra energy will be two sure signs that the Hybrid Diet is working for you. But is there another – more scientific – way to monitor how you are doing in both phases of the diet? Well, yes, there is.

At the most basic level, you will need to measure your glucose (G) and ketone (K) levels, which you can do at any time of the day as you experiment with different foods, combinations and circumstances, such as adding exercise or having an alcoholic drink. In an ideal world, it is also beneficial to know your insulin level, as this rises when your glucose rises, falls when your glucose falls, and is especially low when you are in ketosis. As we saw in Chapter 14, it also plays a key role in switching autophagy (the body's self-repair mechanism) on and off.

Measuring G, K and GKI

If you are in the high fat phase, your principal aim is to reduce your level of glucose and increase your level of ketones. If you are in the slow carb phase, your glucose level (G score) should be between 5 and 6mM both before and two hours after a meal, whereas your goal is about 3mM in the high fat phase. (Don't worry if you don't get there immediately, though; it can take a couple of weeks.)

You will know that you're in mild ketosis when your K score (ketone level) rises above 0.5mM. Thereafter, it may eventually reach 4 or 5mM. You will probably lose weight (and feel great) at anything more than 1mM, but sufferers from epilepsy or brain cancer should try to get their levels as high as possible. We suggest that everyone aim for 3mM.

Since your goal is to keep your glucose down and your ketones up in the high fat phase, it's a good idea to measure the *ratio* between the two. This is called your glucose ketone index (GKI). So, glucose (mM) ÷ ketones (mM) = GKI (see the illustration below).

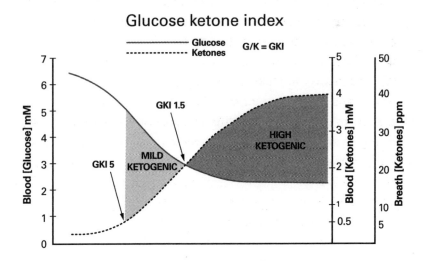

Glucose ketone index

If you start with a healthy blood sugar level of 5mM and a ketone level of 0.5mM, your GKI is 10. You might achieve this in the slow carb phase. Now, if you switch to the high fat phase, your ketone level might increase to 1mM (mild ketosis), while your glucose remains at 5mM, giving a GKI of 5. Keep going, avoiding carbs as much as possible, and your glucose might drop to 4.5mM while your ketone level rises to 1.5mM. You have now hit your target GKI of 3 and are clearly in ketosis.

It's possible to go even further. For instance, if your glucose dropped as low as 2mM and your ketones rose to 4mM, your GKI would be 0.5. This is often the goal for people with epilepsy, diabetes or cancer, because there is evidence that a very low GKI aids the treatment and/or mitigation of all three conditions.[106] However, it is difficult to achieve. If your goal is simply to lose weight and feel great, a GKI of 3 would be absolutely fine.

How to Measure Ketones and Glucose

Ketones can be measured in the blood, breath or urine. As you can see opposite, there are three different kinds: acetoacetate (AcAc), beta-hydroxybutyrate (BHB) and acetone (AC). AcAc is excreted in the urine, so it can be measured using a ketostick, which you pee on; BHB is measured in a pinprick of blood; and AC is excreted in the breath, so it can be measured with a type of breathalyser known as a Ketonix®. All three methods have their merits and drawbacks in terms of ease of use, cost and accuracy. You can see demonstrations of each at www.hybriddiet.co.uk/GKtesting.

How the liver makes ketones

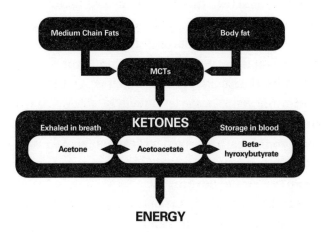

The Ketonix® Breath Test

The Ketonix® breathalyser is probably the easiest and cheapest way to measure ketones. It consists of the measuring device and a rechargeable battery pack. Alternatively, it can be powered through a computer's USB port. The reading is transmitted to, and stored by, an app on a smartphone or computer. The main part of the display is a dial (like a speedometer), with blue, green, yellow and red regions. Blue (0–4 parts per million or ppm) means you are not in ketosis; green (4–30ppm) means you are; and red (above 80ppm) means that your level of ketones is dangerously high.

The system is easy to use (although it takes about ten minutes to reboot if you have unplugged the battery pack). A greater concern is its accuracy, because you can get different readings depending on how you breathe into the tube. Acetone tends to accumulate in the lowest part of the lungs, so aim to blow out every last millilitre of air. Keep exhaling until you are almost gasping. This is hard to do at first, but you'll get used to it, then make sure you use the same technique every time.

Acetone in the breath is a fair reflection of BHB in the blood.

Broadly speaking, assuming you exhale fully, an AC score of 7ppm equates to 1μM of BHB in the blood (see below). So, to calculate your GKI, you will need to divide you Ketonix measurement by seven.

Overall, the major advantage of the Ketonix system is that it provides data on the effects of different foods, meals and circumstances during the high fat phase, which is great information to have at your fingertips because you will be able to see what sends your K score up and down. Moreover, if there is an increase in the ketones in your breath, coupled with a reduction in your level of blood glucose (see below), you will know that what you are doing is working in terms of burning fat.

However, bear in mind that drinking alcohol will send your reading sky high for several hours, because the device is measuring acetone, which is an alcohol. Therefore, you will often get a false reading if you measure your ketones first thing in the morning after consuming alcohol the night before, and certainly if you blow in the tube not long after having a drink. Mouthwash also contains alcohol, so it has a similar impact on the results. Moreover, ironically, a carb-rich diet can generate a falsely high reading. This is because yeast and/or bacteria in the gut can turn the sugar in carbohydrates into alcohol. A classic symptom of this condition would be bloating after eating fruit. Consequently, the Ketonix gives accurate readings only if you are on a low carb, high fat diet, not drinking alcohol and not using mouthwash.

Exercise is another variable. Obviously, your body needs more energy during exercise and it gets it from ketones. Therefore, you will exhale extra acetone in the middle of a long gym session or a halfway through a five-mile run. Wait a few minutes after finishing to get an accurate reading.

Ketosticks

In theory, ketosticks, which are used to measure acetoacetate (AcAc) in the urine, should be the most accurate method of measuring ketones because you pee out acetoacetate whenever you are in ketosis. They are also easy to use and relatively cheap – about ten pence per stick (see Resources). You can either dip the stick in a pot of urine for a few seconds or pee on it midstream until the indicator changes colour. Either way, the measurement will vary depending on when you conduct the test: for instance, it will be higher first thing in the morning or if you are dehydrated after a workout. Therefore, we recommend testing your second pee of the morning and ensuring that you are not dehydrated by drinking sufficient water beforehand.

It can be difficult to determine the exact colour that is registered on the stick, especially in the pink (0.5–1.5µM) and mauve (4–8µM) ranges. The latter, which indicates ketosis, corresponds to about 1–3µM of BHB in the blood.[107] So, to calculate your GKI, think of low mauve (4) as roughly equivalent to a K score of 1, and high mauve (8) as roughly equivalent to a K score of 3. In truth, you can't trust a ketostick to be totally accurate, although it does provide a fairly good visual representation of the journey into ketosis if you compare the results over a few days. Another issue arises once you are in ketogenesis, however, because you tend to excrete less AcAc as time goes by because you are efficiently using up ketones for energy, which may give a false indication that you are no longer in that state.

Measuring Ketones and Glucose in the Blood

Scientific researchers rarely use either breath or urine tests to measure ketone levels because both are considered too imprecise. Instead, they measure the level of beta-hydroxybutyrate (BHB) in a pinprick of blood, as this gives far more accurate results.

If you choose to do the same, the only issue to bear in mind is that your body uses BHB to meet its energy requirements as and when required during ketosis, so a low measurement doesn't necessarily indicate that you have left ketosis. Instead, your body may simply have had unusually high energy demands over the previous few hours (for instance, if you've been for a long run) and has used up the available BHB in your bloodstream. Similarly, a high reading doesn't necessarily indicate that you are in ketosis if your energy demands have been unusually low. For example, if you took a shot of exogenous ketones but were still eating carbs and not exercising, your BHB level will go up – but that doesn't mean you're in ketogenises, burning ketones instead of glucose. So, all we can say is that you are *probably* in ketosis if your score is more than 0.5µM. The best way to eliminate any uncertainty is to measure your blood ketone level two or three times a day. After a week or more on a ketogenic diet, once you're in ketogenesis thus running on ketones, you should expect to have at least 3µM of BHB in your blood.

A high level of breath acetone, a low level of blood BHB and low blood glucose usually indicate that you are burning the fat you eat very efficiently. On the other hand, if you have high BHB and low breath acetone, you are probably good at eating fat but not too great at burning it. In this case, it might be a good idea to start supplementing the hybrid support nutrients (see Chapter 25).

A number of meters are now available that allow you to measure your blood glucose and BHB in the comfort of your own home. Those that use individual ketone and glucose strips range in price from £10 to £25, with the more, expensive versions usually including some of the strips. However, the cost soon adds up when you run out and have to buy more, because each replacement ketone strip can cost anywhere between £1 and £3, depending on the brand. A simpler alternative – and certainly more cost-effective over the long term – is the KEYA® Smart Meter (see Resources), which measures both glucose and ketones after a drop of blood is added to a single strip. The best deal is a package that includes 110 strips – enough for more than three months of daily tests, meaning you can test your daily G and K scores and work out your GKI for as little as a £1.35 a day. By the end of that period, you'll be the master of your metabolism.

Measuring Glucose with the Freestyle Libre Monitor

Recently, you may have noticed a white disc on the arm of Theresa May. This is the sensor of a Freestyle Libre glucose monitor. It allows constant monitoring of blood glucose, is comfortable to wear and supposedly doesn't have to be removed in the bath or shower (although we had one that stopped working after a few lengths in the local swimming pool).

The monitor was designed to help diabetics – such as the Prime Minister, who has type 1 diabetes – to control their blood sugar, but this means that it is also a very useful tool for anyone embarking on the Hybrid Diet. This is because it allows you to see which foods are doing what, and for how long, in either the high fat or the slow carb phase. For instance, as well as seeing a spike after eating a piece of toast, you will be able monitor the impact of adding jam or peanut butter. Given that we are all different, this will help you establish the best foods for your own unique metabolism. You can also view each day's measurements as a graph, and compare these over time.

The Freestyle Libre doesn't actually measure blood glucose level. Rather, it analyses the interstitial fluid that surrounds the cells beneath your skin. This provides an accurate reflection of blood glucose,[108] but there is a lag of about five to ten minutes.[109] Otherwise, we have found that it correlates very well with the KEYA® pinprick monitor. The whole system consists of the reader, which is inexpensive and easy to use, and the sensor, which has a very thin pin that is pushed painlessly into the arm with an applicator. Unfortunately, though, the sensor lasts only two weeks and each one currently costs £50!

Your GP might be able to prescribe both the reader and the sensors on the NHS if you have diabetes, or you could simply buy them online if you don't (see Resources). It might be worth the investment, as you will certainly learn a lot about your metabolism and could well lower your glucose and HbA1c levels as a result.

Your Ideal Blood Glucose Level

Your blood glucose should remain relatively stable throughout the day, without any large peaks or troughs, although it will obviously rise whenever you eat carbs, then decline as your insulin kicks in. Before eating, your glucose level should be in the range of 4–5.5µM. After eating, it might rise (ideally gradually) to 8µM within the first thirty minutes, but it should never go above 9µM. Two hours later, if everything is working well, your so-called 'post-prandial blood sugar' should have returned to its starting point. If it remains high – above 6.5µM – that's an indicator of diabetes.

If your blood sugar rises too high, and/or too fast, your arteries, eyes and kidneys suffer wear and tear, and your whole body is more likely to suffer inflammation. It will also have little or no opportunity to repair itself during autophagy.

During ketosis, blood glucose can drop below 3µM. We have even recorded a level that was closer to 2µM! Under normal circumstances, this would be considered very bad news – a sure sign of a dangerous condition called hypoglycaemia. However, studies have shown that the body and brain can continue to function perfectly well with extremely low levels of glucose in the blood because it can meet almost all of its energy needs from ketones. Nevertheless, we do not recommend trying to force your blood glucose below 2µM.

Your Ideal Glycosylated Haemoglobin Level

A high level of glycosylated haemoglobin in the blood is the best long-term indicator of problems with blood sugar control.

It is tested by measuring HbA1c, which is below 5.6 per cent (or 37mmol/mol) in a healthy body. The table below shows how to interpret HbA1c results.

Healthy	Not great	Dysglycemia	Diabetes
<5.6%	5.6–6.5%	>6.5%	>7%
<37mmol/mol	37–48mmol/mol	>49mmol/mol	>53mmol/mol

Your doctor will conduct this test if they are concerned that you might have diabetes, or it might be included in a more advanced blood 'work up'. Red blood cells (haemoglobin) live for about three months, and if they are glycosylated (effectively coated with sugar), they remain that way. So, a high percentage of glycosylated red blood cells indicates a high number of sugar spikes over the previous three-month period. If your glycosylated haemoglobin is more than 7 per cent (53mmol/mol), the chances are that you already have diabetes or will soon develop it.

Unlike glucose, your level of HbA1c does not change overnight, which makes it a much more accurate indicator of diabetes. However, this also means that it takes a while to see any significant improvement after altering your diet. And it will be three months before you see the full effect.

You can measure your own HbA1c at home (see Resources). We recommend doing this before starting the Hybrid Diet and then three months later. You can also help yourself – and others – by completing the online 100% Health questionnaire at www.patrickholford.com, in which we ask for both of these scores.

Although HbA1c is a very valuable and informative test, it will not tell you if or when you have entered ketosis in the high fat phase. For that, you will need to conduct a blood, urine or breath analysis of your ketone levels, as described above.

Glucose and Ketone Monitoring in Action

A short video at www.holforddiet.co.uk/GKtesting shows how all of the monitors described in this chapter work.

To recap, you will know that you are in full-blown ketosis when your blood BHB reaches 3μM *or* your breath acetone reaches the green zone (30ppm) *or* your urine acetoacetate level reaches 8μM. When you reach any of these levels, your blood glucose is likely to be around 3μM and certainly less than 5μM. If your blood BHB is more than 1μM, breath AC more than 10ppm or ketostick reading 'moderate 4', we would term this 'mild ketosis'.

After testing all three for several days, we found that dividing breath acetone (in ppm) by seven gives a rough approximation of blood BHB (in μM). So, if you get a reading of 21ppm from the breathalyser test, you can assume that you have about 3μM of BHB in your blood (i.e. you are in ketosis). Meanwhile, we found that ketosticks give results that are slightly more than double those in the pinprick test. For example, you need to be in the region of 'high 8' before you can assume that your blood BHB is 3μM.

G and K scores during baseline and high fat and slow carb weeks

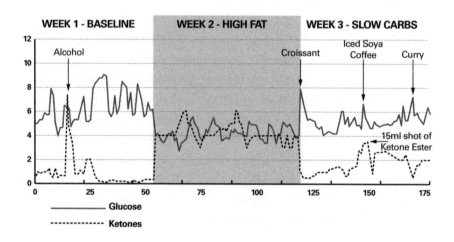

For simplicity, it makes sense to convert breath or urine tests into blood BHB on the basis of these guidelines.

I (Patrick) measured the acetone in my breath (which I then converted into blood BHB by dividing by seven) and my blood glucose throughout a 'baseline' week, a high fat week and a slow carb week. The results are presented opposite.

During the baseline week, I ate my usual, reasonably healthy, lowish GL diet. The really big spike in the K score was caused by a glass of alcohol, so it is a false reading. (Remember, the Ketonix breathalyser cannot distinguish between alcohol and ketones.) Otherwise, as you can see, my ketone score remained pretty stable and generally below 1μM. Meanwhile, my G score was healthy because the average was slightly less than 5μM in the dips between meals.

I kickstarted the high fat phase with a thirty-minute run to burn off some glycogen and finished dinner at 6 p.m., so I achieved a sixteen-hour fast before my first high fat breakfast at 10 a.m. Following that, my G score was right down while my K score was around 4μM. Thereafter, both scores remained fairly stable throughout the week, with the troughs of the G score averaging around 4μM. In other trials, when I have continued in the high fat phase for up to three weeks, my G score has dropped to between 2 and 3μM – an indication that I have switched into full-blown ketosis. (Note that this would be a cause for concern for someone who was not on a strict ketogenic diet, and an indication of hypo for type 1 diabetic.)

I had a croissant just before starting the slow carb phase, which caused my G score to shoot up as I exited ketosis almost immediately. The next spike was an iced soya coffee from Starbucks. Then, towards the end of the week, I went out for a curry. I chose carefully and avoided bread and rice. Instead, I had half a poppadum, some dahl and a prawn balit, but my blood sugar still spiked to more than 7μM. Overall, though, the G scores in the final week remained in a tighter and lower band than they had been in the first week. Halfway through, as an experiment, I had a 15ml shot of ketone ester, which generated a significant spike in my K score.

Precise Monitoring

After that three-week 'warm-up', it was time to assess the high fat and slow carb phases in fine detail. I followed the prescribed daily menus on page 232 for three days, then the prescribed menus on page 258 for three days (with one or two slight variations). I measured glucose and ketone levels thirty minutes after starting each meal, then the glucose level two hours after finishing each meal. Of course, this meant I could then calculate my GKI.

G, K and GKI scores over the course of three high fat days

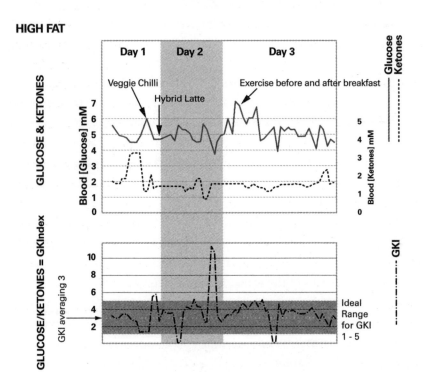

The chart above shows the effect of starting the high fat phase with a fifteen-hour fast between the previous night's dinner and Day 1's breakfast. I was already 'fat adapted' (on account of the three-week warm-up), so my K score increased rapidly. The vegetable chilli in the evening of Day 1 pushed up my G score, but it soon fell back down to base level. Day 2 started very well with a Hybrid Latté, which we have found consistently lowers G and raises K, and the rest of the day was good, too. The G score spike on Day 3 was due to exercising. Glucose is liberated from the body's reserves of glycogen when the muscles need more than usual, and thereafter it can be a couple of hours before blood sugar settles down again. By the end of Day 3, my K score was between 1.5 and 2μM (mild ketosis), while my G score was steady at around 4μM. My GKI was right in the middle of the ideal range at about 3.

This brief experiment revealed that the quickest way to enter ketosis is to fast, either completely, for a day or two, or for fourteen to sixteen hours (early dinner, late breakfast), then drink a Hybrid Latté for your Day 1 breakfast, then avoid all carbs (except those that are in green vegetables) throughout the rest of the day and into Day 2.

Next, I switched to three days of slow carbs (see overleaf).

I started Day 1 with a Get Up & Go shake with some berries, then had an apple and some nuts as a mid-morning snack, followed by a big bowl of Chestnut and Butter Bean Soup for lunch, then a late afternoon snack. As you can see from the chart above, my G score increased to more than 7μM after each meal or snack, but soon fell back down to about 6. The evening meal had quite a low glycemic load (8 GL), so my G score peaked at just 6.5 before falling to less than 5 by late evening, where it presumably remained throughout the night. (I did not conduct any measurements during the night).

I started Day 2 with a quite low G score of 4.8μM. Coffee brought it up to 5.7, then I had chia and oat porridge with berries before a half-hour cycle ride through London. This combination of food and exercise generated a peak of 9, but my G score soon fell

G, K and GKI scores over the course of three slow carb days

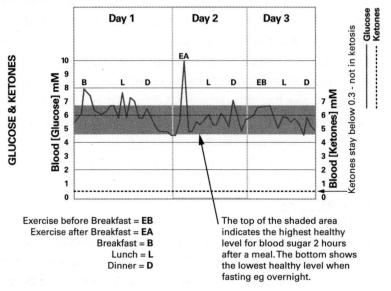

SLOW CARB

Exercise before Breakfast = **EB**
Exercise after Breakfast = **EA**
Breakfast = **B**
Lunch = **L**
Dinner = **D**

The top of the shaded area indicates the highest healthy level for blood sugar 2 hours after a meal. The bottom shows the lowest healthy level when fasting eg overnight.

back to 5 and stayed there even after a mid-morning snack. I went off-piste at lunchtime by eating out. The delicious meal consisted of a mushroom starter followed by tempura haddock with cauliflower cheese and peas, plus a glass of Chardonnay. Nevertheless, by 3 p.m., my G score was just 6 and falling. I had a slice of Apple and Almond Cake when I got home, which pushed it back up to 6. After dinner, it peaked at 7, but it was back below 5 by 11 p.m.

On Day 3 I went for a half-hour run before breakfast, which helped to push my G score up to 6.7µM, but by midday it was back down to 5. It peaked at just 5.9 after lunch, then again after a slice of Carrot and Walnut Cake at 4 p.m. But thereafter it steadily declined to 4.7 before dinner at 8 p.m., which I enjoyed with a glass of white wine. (You can allow yourself the occasional drink or dessert during the slow carb phase.) By 10 p.m., I was back below 5.

As you can see from my result in the chart above, I was

nowhere near ketosis throughout this three-day slow carb phase, whereas my blood sugar level undulated like a range of small hills. This sort of response to food indicates that the body is not secreting large amounts of insulin production, little glycosylation is occurring in the blood, and no sugar is being converted to fat for storage. My blood sugar remained very stable throughout, although the average reading was rather lower on Day 3 than Day 1 because by then I had become 'carb adapted'. If a diabetic were to achieve these results over a somewhat longer period of time, they could abandon their medication, as they would no longer be classified as having diabetes.

The Results

So, what did following the Hybrid Diet for four weeks do for me? Well, at the start of the 'warm-up' period, I weighed 12 stones (76kg). By the end of the second slow carb phase, I weighed 10 stones 6lb (66kg) – roughly the weight I was in my twenties. And this was achieved without any change to my exercise routine.

Remember, you will lose 4 or 5lb (2kg) of fluid from your body at the start of the high fat phase, then put it back on as soon as you begin the slow carb phase, so factor this in if you weigh yourself on those days. However, you will lose roughly equal amounts of *real* weight (i.e. fat) in each of the two phases of the Hybrid Diet. If you follow our guidelines and don't have too many lapses, you can expect to lose about 4lb (2kg) each week – that is, more than a stone in a month.

Part 5

Hybrid Diet Menus and Recipes

To help you put the Hybrid Diet principles into practice, we have compiled enough recipes for you to choose a week's worth for each of the high fat and slow carb phases, plus extra ideas to help you stick to the diet when cooking your own dishes or eating out. Most of the recipes have been adapted from Patrick's *Low GL Diet Bible*, *The Low GL Diet Cookbook* or *Ten Secrets of 100% Health Cookbook*, so we are deeply indebted to Patrick's wonderful 'kitchen wizard' – Fiona McDonald Joyce – who trained at the Institute for Optimum Nutrition and knows how to devise delicious dishes that follow all of the guidelines contained within this book. We have built up a library of terrific recipes over the last ten years, many of which can be prepared incredibly quickly. Others could be served at any dinner party and receive five-star ratings without the guests ever realising they were eating something super-healthy.

A few simple adaptations – such as using chicken thighs with the skin on rather than skinless chicken breast, or oily mackerel instead of haddock, or adding a spoonful of tahini – can turn most of the slow carb recipes (which are designed to deliver a total of 40 GLs a day) into high fat recipes (which meet the daily fat requirement and keep the carbs below 15 GLs).

Chapter 27

High Fat Phase Breakfasts, Snacks, Lunches and Dinners

All the breakfasts, main meals and snacks are designed to give you 10 FUs (fat units) and no more than 15 GLs a day – the daily allowance of carbs if you are to remain in ketosis. As three tablespoons of C8 MCT oil (3 FUs) is one of the most direct ways to generate ketones, we have included this each day, so the food itself provides only 7 FUs. Note that we rate a 10ml shot of exogenous ketones (see Resources) or two servings of ketone salts as 1 FU, so you could use these instead of the C8 oil if you prefer.

We give the number of carbs for each recipe and as a daily total. The recipes and daily menus are also designed to give you all the protein you need, but not too much.

While anything less than 15 GLs of carbs should see you entering and remaining in ketosis, we are all different, so you might find a combination of intermittent fasting and even lower carbs – less than 10 GLs – help you enter ketosis more rapidly. We have assumed that you will fast for fifteen hours between dinner and breakfast on the first few days, and that you will give yourself an energy boost with one coffee in the morning. The latter will help you to stave off any hunger pangs. However, it should be remembered that caffeine gives you energy like a bank loan gives you wealth. Once you are in ketosis, it's better to quit the caffeine, and there's no need to fast as you are now in the keto zone.

We also recommend supplements (see Chapter 25), especially carnitine, which helps the body to burn both fat and ketones.

Breakfasts

Hybrid Latté (page 305)
Scrambled Egg with Smoked Salmon and Avocado (page 306)
Salmon with Asparagus Omelette (page 307)
Bacon (or pork or salmon) with scrambled eggs
Chia or Walnut Coconut Yoghurt with Blueberries or Strawberries (page 308)

Snacks

Taramasalata with crudités – celery or cucumber sticks
½ avocado with ½ tablespoon of tahini or Guacamolé (page 308) with crudités
Goat's cheese with small handful of walnuts
Goat's Cheese and Artichoke Paté (see page 309)
Hummus and Egg Paté (page 309)
Gravadlax with Quail's Eggs (page 310)

Main Meals

Marinated Salmon Steak with Sautéed Pesto Greens (page 310)
Low Carb Kedgeree (page 311)
Hummus Soufflé (page 313)
Bangers and Cauliflower Mash (page 314)
Spiced Turkey Burgers (page 314)
Nick's Beefburgers (page 315)
Rib-eye Steak (page 316) with Broccoli and Cauliflower Mash (see page 324)
Vegetarian Chilli (page 316)
Chilli con Carne (page 317)
Roasted Pepper Rolls with Goat's Cheese and Pine Nut Stuffing (page 319)
Chicken Curry (page 320)
Pork Medallions with Watercress Salsa Verde (page 321)
Smoked Salmon with Crème Fraîche and Herb Sauce (page 322)
Creamy Salmon with Leeks (page 322)
Cauliflower, Chickpea and Egg Curry (page 323)
Cauliflower Mash (page 324)
Cauliflower Rice (page 325)

Recipes

Breakfasts

Hybrid Latté

This is a great morning kickstart, free from carbs, rich in ketone-friendly fats and both tasty and filling. It's good hot and, by adding ice into the blender, also works as an iced latté. Serves 1.

240ml (8fl oz) low carb almond milk (unsweetened)
120ml (4fl oz) filtered coffee or run through (less caffeine, more antioxidants)
1 heaped tbsp almond butter or peanut butter (almond has half the carbs)
1 tbsp walnuts, pecans or peanuts
1 tbsp C8 oil with carnitine (Ketofast)
1 rounded tsp cacao powder
½ tsp cinnamon (good for blood sugar)

Blend all ingredients in a blender.

Note: Leave out the coffee for caffeine free, or use decaf and add more almond milk and a cup of ice cubes for an iced version.
3 FU, 2 GL/8g carbs

Scrambled Egg with Smoked Salmon and Avocado

Easy to put together on a busy morning, this filling breakfast is low GL but full of fats to fuel the brain. Serves 1.

2 eggs
Butter or olive oil
1 slice smoked salmon
½ avocado
1 rough oatcake

Whisk the eggs, season and scramble over a medium heat with the butter and oil. Serve with the remaining ingredients.
2 FU, 2 GL/6g carbs

Salmon with Asparagus Omelette

This dish ticks a lot of boxes, with the oily fish and egg providing brain-friendly fats and the green vegetables adding fibre and vitamins. You can adapt this recipe according to personal taste or what you have in the fridge: try steamed spinach or perhaps stir-fried shiitake mushrooms as an omelette filling. Serves 1.

3 free range or organic eggs
Pinch of sea salt
50g (2oz) fine asparagus spears, trimmed
Knob of butter, ghee or coconut oil
1 heaped tbsp diced smoked salmon (more if desired)
Freshly ground black pepper
Wedge of lemon

1   Beat the eggs and salt together in a bowl.
2   Put the asparagus on to steam for around 5 minutes or until *al dente*. Ensure that you take it off the heat as soon as it is cooked. While this is cooking, make the omelette.
3   Heat a small frying pan over a medium heat, add the butter or oil and move it around the pan to coat the base and sides, then pour in the eggs.
4   When the base has coloured and set, place the asparagus over half of the omelette and top with the smoked salmon. Sprinkle with black pepper, then carefully fold in half and let sit for half a minute to cook the middle. Serve immediately with a wedge of lemon.

Note: Gluten-, wheat-, dairy- (if using oil) and yeast-free.
2 FU, 1 GL/2g carbs

Chia or Walnut Coconut Yoghurt with Blueberries or Strawberries

This tasty combo provides protein, good fats and antioxidants. It's good for breakfast or a snack. Serves 1.

100g (3½oz) coconut yoghurt
1 tbsp chia seeds or chopped walnuts
Handful of berries

Mix the yoghurt with the chia seeds and berries and serve.
2 FU, 1.5 GL/7.8g carbs

Snacks

Guacamole

Fresh chilli, garlic and spring onions give this version of the Mexican speciality a real kick. It is easy to make in a few minutes. Makes 2 servings.

1 ripe avocado
Juice of ½ a lime
2 cloves of garlic, crushed
1 tbsp finely chopped fresh coriander
4 spring onions, finely chopped
¼ mild chilli, deseeded
Freshly ground black pepper

Mash all of the ingredients together and adjust the seasoning according to taste.
1 FU, 1 GL/2g carbs

Goat's Cheese and Artichoke Pâté

Creamy goat's cheese complements the subtle flavour of artichoke. This remarkable vegetable (which is a member of the thistle family) is very good for the liver and can boost detoxification. Makes 2 servings.

50g (2oz) marinated artichoke hearts in oil, drained
50g (2oz) mild soft goat's cheese
Freshly ground black pepper

Mash all of the ingredients together.
1 FU, 3 GL/7g carbs

Hummus and Egg Pâté

Egg mayo gets a makeover here, using hummus for a rich flavour. Use ready-made hummus as it has a smoother, softer consistency than homemade. This can be stored in the fridge for up to three days. Makes 2 servings.

2 eggs, hard boiled for 8 minutes, shelled
100g (3½oz) hummus
½ tbsp finely chopped fresh flat leaf parsley
Freshly ground black pepper

1   Mash the eggs into the hummus.
2   Add the parsley and black pepper, then mix everything together.
1 FU, 1 GL/4g carbs

Gravadlax with Quail's Eggs

Gravadlax is smoked salmon cured with dill and other herbs, which gives the fish an intense, zesty flavour. Look for a brand that doesn't contain sugar – or make your own. This dish is also packed with nutrients, from the omega-3 fats in the salmon to the zinc in the eggs. Here, we pair it with quail's eggs for a light snack. Serves 2.

100g (3½oz) gravadlax slices
5cm (2in) chunk of cucumber, peeled and deseeded, then grated into ribbons or julienned
4 quail's eggs, hardboiled for 4 minutes, peeled and halved
2 tsp lemon juice
Freshly ground black pepper

1   Arrange the gravadlax slices in a nest in the middle of each plate.
2   Place the cucumber strips within the nests and arrange the quail's egg halves in the middle of each nest.
3   Drizzle each dish with lemon juice and sprinkle with black pepper before serving.

1 FU, 0 GL/1.3g carbs

Main Meals

Marinated Salmon Steak with Sautéed Pesto Greens

This is a simple midweek meal that's delicious too. Serves 1.

Spice marinade:

4 tbsp olive oil
½ tsp whole-grain mustard
Juice of 1 lemon

½ tsp cumin
½ tsp ground coriander

1 salmon steak
100–150g (3½–5¼oz) spinach and/or kale
1 tbsp ghee or butter or coconut butter
50g (2oz) basil pesto (we like the dairy free Happy Pear brand or make your own with fresh basil leaves, ground pine nuts, olive oil and Parmesan)

1   Mix the marinade ingredients together to taste and pour over the top and sides of the salmon steak, with the skin side down. Leave for 15 minutes to soak in.
2   Place the salmon in pre-heated oven at 180°C/350°F for 10 minutes.
3   Melt a tablespoon of ghee in a wide frying pan with a lid (use a steam fry pan if you have one), stir in the greens and add the pesto. Turn the heat down to low, cover and leave to cook for 3 minutes.

2 FU, 1 GL/4g carbs

Low Carb Kedgeree

By using mackerel instead of the traditional haddock, creamed with a tablespoon of tahini, and a small serving of Kamut bulgur instead of rice, this spicy kedgeree is both high in fat and low GL. Serves 4.

60g (2oz) Kamut bulgur, which makes 180g cooked (or red lentils to lower the GL)
2 free range or organic eggs
2 tbsp mild, medium (not extra virgin) olive oil, virgin rapeseed oil or coconut oil
1 clove of garlic, crushed

1 large or 2 small onions, finely chopped
½–1 tsp ground smoked paprika or cayenne (depending on how hot you like it)
½–1 tsp ground cumin
½–1 tsp ground turmeric
2 smoked mackerel fillets
200g (7oz) Tenderstem broccoli
100g (3½oz) frozen petit pois
Salt and freshly ground black pepper
1 tbsp tahini
4 tbsp finely chopped flat leaf parsley

1 Measure out three times as much water as Kamut bulgur by volume and bring to the boil. Add the Kamut bulgur and simmer for 8 minutes, then drain any surplus water. (If you time it right and use the right amount of water, there'll be no need to drain.)

2 Hard boil the eggs in a pan of boiling water for 6 minutes, cool them rapidly under the tap for a minute, then set aside to cool fully before peeling and slicing into quarters.

3 Add the olive oil to a large saucepan and sweat the garlic and onion for a minute or so before adding the spices. Let them gently cook for a further few minutes until the onions are soft and fragrant, taking care not to let them burn.

4 Break the smoked mackerel into small pieces and add to the saucepan, stirring them in.

5 Add the frozen petit pois to boiling water and wait until the water is boiling again, then add the broccoli. Once the peas float to the top, drain off the water.

6 Stir the cooked Kamut bulgur into the onion and spice mixture until evenly coated. Add the cooked peas, broccoli florets and eggs. Season and serve.

7   Add the tahini to make it creamy and season with plenty
    of pepper. You won't need any salt due to the salt in the fish
    and the strength of the spices.
8   Add the parsley as a garnish.

1 FU, 4 GL/17g carbs

Hummus Soufflé

This recipe is so simple but it makes for an impressive-looking,
tasty starter that will help you to stay in ketosis. The beaten egg
whites hold the mixture in a classic soufflé shape before you even
cook it, meaning there is none of the usual angst of waiting for
the soufflé to rise. Use ready-made hummus, as its soft consistency
works better than the coarser homemade variety. Serves 2.

1 tbsp mixed pepper antipasto in oil, drained
1 tbsp finely chopped fresh flat leaf parsley
100g (3½oz) hummus
2 medium egg whites

1   Preheat the oven to 190°C/375°F.
2   Cut the pepper antipasto into strips and place in the bottom
    of two ramekins.
3   Stir the parsley into the hummus.
4   Beat the egg whites until they form stiff peaks.
5   Gently fold the egg into the hummus using a metal spoon
    and carefully spoon into the ramekins, making a mountain
    shape on top like a risen soufflé.
6   Bake for 15 minutes.

1 FU, 5 GL/ 5g carb

Bangers and Cauliflower Mash

There's nothing quite like a plate of good quality sausages and mash. As potatoes are very high GL, we recommend our thick, comforting cauliflower mash instead. Serves 2.

4 good quality, pork sausages (preferably rare breed, free range, vaccine and antibiotic free, such as those at www.forestcoalpitfarm.co.uk)
2 portions of Cauliflower Mash (page 324)

1   Cook the sausages according to the pack instructions (grill or oven cook rather than fry to reduce the fat content).
2   Meanwhile, make the cauliflower mash.
3   Serve with the cooked sausages.
2 FU, 5 GL/6.5g carbs

Spiced Turkey Burgers

The alternative burger. Turkey mince is much leaner than pork, beef or lamb, and the garlic, chilli and spices give these burgers a terrific kick. They're great served with cauliflower mash. Serves 2.

250g (9oz) turkey mince
1 egg yolk, beaten
4 spring onions, finely chopped
1 mild red chilli, deseeded and pith removed
2 cloves of garlic, crushed
½ tsp ground cumin
½ tsp ground coriander
Salt and freshly ground black pepper
2 portions of Cauliflower Mash (page 324)

1   Mix the turkey mince with the rest of the ingredients, except the mash, season and leave to sit in the fridge to marinate for at least an hour.
2   Shape into burgers and grill under a medium heat for 10 minutes, then turn and grill for a further 7 minutes.
3   Meanwhile, make the cauliflower mash (see page 324).
4   Season to taste and serve with the burgers

2 FU, 5 GL/4g carbs (including the mash)

Nick's Beefburgers

These delicious burgers can be made in advance and chilled until you are ready to cook them. Cauliflower mash makes a great accompaniment. Serves 2.

1 tbsp tamari or soy sauce
1 tsp Worcestershire sauce
1 tbsp finely chopped fresh coriander
¼ red onion, finely chopped
½ egg, beaten
½ tsp sea salt
½ tsp black pepper
200g (7oz) extra lean beef mince
2 portions of Cauliflower Mash (page 324)

1   Mix together everything aside from the mince (and cauliflower), then add to the mince and knead well to mix.
2   Divide into four patties and flatten each into a burger. Place on a plate, cover and put in the fridge to firm up for approximately 10 minutes, or until required.
3   Grill the burgers under a medium heat for approximately 7 minutes per side (or to taste, but do not burn).

4 Meanwhile, make the cauliflower mash. Season to taste and
   serve with the burgers.
2 FU, 5 GL/ 4g carb (includes the mash)

Rib-eye Steak

Rib-eye steak is a fatty cut of meat, and you increase FUs by
searing it with butter. This is another recipe that's great with
cauliflower mash. Serves 1.

100g (4oz) of rib-eye steak – this is a high fat cut
Knob of butter
Pinch of salt
Finely ground black pepper
1 portion Cauliflower Mash (page 324)

1 Season the steak, then sear on both sides for 5 minutes in a
   frying pan with the butter.
2 Transfer to a preheated oven, 180°C/350°F, and roast for
   30 minutes.
3 Meanwhile, make the cauliflower mash. Season to taste
   and serve.
2 FU, 5 GL/4g carbs (includes the mash)

Vegetarian Chilli

Packed with beans, vegetables and spices, this hearty vegetarian chilli carries plenty of heat. It keeps in the fridge for up to
three days (which will enhance the flavour) and freezes well,
too. Cauliflower rice (page 325) is a great accompaniment to this
chilli. Pinto and/or black-eye beans work just as well as kidney
and borlotti. Serves 4.

2 tsp coconut oil or olive oil

1 onion, diced

2 cloves of garlic, crushed

1 pepper, diced

1 tsp ground cumin

1 tsp crushed chilli flakes

1 tsp chilli powder

250g (9oz) mushrooms, sliced

400g (14oz) can chopped tomatoes

3 tbsp tomato purée

410g (14¼oz) can kidney beans, rinsed and drained

410g (14¼oz) can borlotti beans, rinsed and drained

3 tsp reduced salt vegetable bouillon powder

1   Heat the oil in a pan and fry the onion and garlic for
    2 minutes.
2   Add the pepper and spices and cover to sweat for 5 minutes,
    until the peppers soften.
3   Add the mushrooms and cook for a few minutes until
    they soften.
4   Tip in the canned tomatoes, tomato purée, beans and
    bouillon powder, then stir thoroughly. Cover and simmer
    for 5 minutes before serving.

2 FU, 6 GL/15g carbs

Chilli con Carne

We recommend making this hot and spicy favourite in advance to allow the flavours to develop. Cook it, cool it, pop it into the fridge and have it the next evening as an easy supper – just heat through and serve. Our version uses more vegetables than standard recipes to optimise the nutrient content. Cauliflower Rice (page 325) is a great accompaniment to this dish. Do not substitute kidney beans for the borlotti/pinto beans as this will push the GL too high. Serves 4.

450g (1lb) lean organic beef mince
2 tsp coconut oil or olive oil
1 onion, diced
2 cloves of garlic, crushed
1 pepper, diced
2 tsp ground cumin
1 tsp chilli powder
1–2 tsp crushed chilli flakes (according to taste)
250g (9oz) mushrooms, sliced
400g (14oz) can chopped tomatoes
3 tbsp tomato purée
4 tsp reduced salt vegetable bouillon powder
410g (14¼oz) can borlotti or pinto beans, rinsed and drained
Freshly ground black pepper

1   Cook the mince in a large frying pan until it starts to brown, scooping off any fat that appears with a teaspoon. Remove the mince and set aside.
2   Heat the oil in the pan and fry the onion, garlic and pepper for a couple of minutes.
3   Add the cumin, chilli powder and chilli flakes to the pan with the vegetables and cook for 10 minutes or so.
4   Add the mushrooms to the pan and cook for a further 5 minutes, until soft.
5   Return the mince to the pan along with the chopped tomatoes, tomato purée, bouillon powder and beans.
6   Cover and simmer for 10–15 minutes, until the vegetables are soft and the flavours have mingled. Season with black pepper to serve.

1 FU, 5 GL/8g carbs

Roasted Pepper Rolls with Goat's Cheese and Pine Nut Stuffing

A full-flavoured dish that can also be served as a starter or a snack, if you half the serving size. It keeps well in the fridge for up to three days. Serves 2.

300g (10½oz) large roasted red peppers, in halves or large pieces
2 tsp lemon juice
100g (3½oz) soft goat's cheese
Freshly ground black pepper
40g (1½oz) pine nuts
1 tbsp finely chopped fresh basil leaves

1   If using home-roasted peppers, slit them up one side, open out and pat dry with some kitchen towels. If using jarred or deli peppers in oil, use the largest pieces you can find and flatten them.
2   Mix the lemon juice with the goat's cheese to loosen it up slightly. Season well with black pepper and stir in the pine nuts and basil.
3   Divide the goat's cheese mixture between the peppers and spread along the middle of each, lengthways.
4   Roll each pepper up to form a cylinder with the goat's cheese filling in the centre, then press between your fingers to stop it from unrolling. Serve immediately or chill.

2 FU, 5 GL/12g carbs

Chicken Curry

Curry nights are not out of bounds during the Hybrid Diet. Coconut milk and immune-boosting spices make this delicious version creamy yet piquant. It will keep in the fridge for up to three days and freezes well, too. Serves 2.

1 tbsp coconut oil or olive oil
2 chicken breasts, sliced into strips
1 tsp ground cumin
½ tsp turmeric
4 cloves of garlic, crushed
1 mild red chilli, deseeded and finely chopped
2 onions, chopped
2 tsp reduced salt vegetable bouillon powder dissolved in 210ml (8fl oz) water
210ml (8fl oz) coconut milk

1   Heat the oil in a frying pan or wok and sear the chicken on both sides, then remove from the pan and set to one side.
2   Fry the cumin and turmeric in the pan for a few seconds before adding the garlic and chilli and sautéing for 30 seconds.
3   Add the onion and fry to soften.
4   Pour the bouillon liquid into the pan with the coconut milk, return the meat to the pan and simmer until the chicken is fully cooked – about 20–30 minutes.

2 FU, 3 GL/2g carbs

Pork Medallions with Watercress Salsa Verde

A great alternative to chicken or fish, the pork is paired with a sharp, herby salsa verde for a kick of fresh flavour and a surge of phytonutrients. This recipe provides enough salsa verde for four servings, so you can use the remainder the next day with fish or mix it with beans to make a delicious salad. It also keeps for up to five days in the fridge. Serves 2.

2 pork medallions
1 clove of garlic, crushed
4 anchovy fillets, drained
1 tbsp capers, rinsed to remove the vinegar and drained
2 tbsp fresh flat leaf parsley
1 tbsp fresh basil leaves
Good handful of watercress, roughly chopped
Freshly ground black pepper
2 tbsp extra virgin olive oil
1 tbsp lemon juice

1   Preheat the grill to a moderate heat and grill the medallions for 15 minutes (or until properly cooked), turning halfway.
2   Meanwhile, make the salsa verde. Place all of the remaining ingredients in a food processor and blitz until the sauce is well combined. Alternatively, you can do this by hand, chopping everything very finely and mixing together thoroughly.
3   Add a dollop of the salsa to each medallion and serve.
2 FU, 3GL/2g carbs

Smoked Salmon with Crème Fraîche and Herb Sauce

This dish is ridiculously easy to make for a speedy supper. The tart crème fraîche contrasts beautifully with the smoky fish. Serves 2.

2 smoked salmon fillets
2 tbsp crème fraîche
1 tbsp of finely chopped flat-leaf parsley
Freshly ground black pepper and salt

1   Gently heat the fish according to the pack instructions.
2   Meanwhile, make the sauce by gently heating the crème fraiche and stirring in the chopped parsley and salt and black pepper to taste.
3   Pour the sauce over the fish and season with a little more black pepper if necessary.

2 FU, 4 GL/3g carbs

Creamy Salmon with Leeks

This is real comfort food, with a wonderfully creamy sauce. It also packs a substantial nutritional punch from the omega-3s and green veg as well as plenty of fibre from the butter beans. Serves 2.

2 tsp coconut oil or olive oil
2 courgettes, thinly sliced horizontally
4 leeks, thinly sliced horizontally
75g (2¾oz) creamy soft goat's cheese
210ml (8fl oz) full fat milk, soya milk or almond milk
2 tbsp cornflour
410g (14¼oz) can butter beans, rinsed and drained
100g (3½oz) smoked salmon, torn into strips
4 spring onions, finely sliced diagonally
2 tsp dill, chopped

1 Heat the oil in a large frying pan or wok and sauté the courgettes and leeks until they start to soften and colour.
2 Add the goat's cheese and half the milk and stir while the cheese melts.
3 Mix the cornflour with the rest of the milk to form a smooth liquid and add to the pan, stirring constantly to avoid any lumps as the sauce thickens.
4 Tip in the drained butter beans, smoked salmon, spring onions and dill, and heat through.

2 FU, 8 GL/18g carbs

Cauliflower, Chickpea and Egg Curry

The chickpeas provide a welcome boost of B vitamins in this delicious dish. Hard boil the eggs before you start cooking. Indeed, the whole curry can be made in advance and then heated through when needed. Serves 4.

3 tbsp coconut oil or virgin rapeseed oil
1 red onion, diced
1 clove of garlic, crushed
Thumb-sized piece of root ginger, peeled and grated
2 tbsp curry paste
1 cauliflower, broken into florets
410g (14¼oz) can chickpeas, rinsed and drained
400ml (14fl oz) coconut milk
4 hard-boiled eggs, peeled and halved lengthways
2 tbsp toasted flaked almonds (optional)
Good handful of roughly chopped fresh coriander
Pinch of salt

1 Heat a wok over a low heat, add the oil, swirl to coat, then stir in the onion and stir fry for around 4 minutes to soften.
2 Add the garlic and ginger and cook for a minute.

3   Stir in the curry paste and cook for a further minute before adding the cauliflower, then stir fry to coat.

4   Add the chickpeas then pour in the coconut milk. Stir and bring to the boil, then reduce the heat, cover the pan and let it simmer for 20–25 minutes, stirring often, or until the sauce is thick and the cauliflower tender. Season to taste.

5   Place the eggs in the curry, half burying them yolk side up, and allow them to warm through for a minute or two before sprinkling the toasted flaked almonds and coriander on top.

2 FU, 9 GL/18g carbs

Cauliflower Mash

This can be used in place of mashed potato in any meal. Broccoli can be used in place of cauliflower if this is more to your taste. Serves 1.

200g (7oz) cauliflower florets
Knob of butter, ghee or olive oil
Parmesan cheese (optional)
Finely ground black pepper

1   Add the cauliflower florets to a pot of boiling water and cook for 7 minutes or until they start to soften. Drain off the water.

2   Mash by hand or put in a blender with butter and (optional) Parmesan cheese. Season with pepper.

1 FU, 1 GL/5g carbs

Cauliflower Rice

This dish can be used in place of rice in any meal. Serves 1.

200g (7oz) cauliflower florets
Drizzle of olive oil

1   If you have a food blender, pulse the cauliflower until
    it resembles grains of rice. If not, use the largest holes
    in a grater.
2   Toss the rice in a drizzle of olive oil.
3   Place in a pre-heated oven at 200°C/4000°F for 12 minutes
    and stir halfway through to disperse the oil. If you prefer,
    the rice can be stir fried for 5 minutes or microwaved on
    high in a bowl covered with cling-film for 2 minutes.
1 FU, 1 GL/5g carbs

Chapter 28

Slow Carb Breakfasts, Snacks, Lunches and Dinners

All the main meals in this chapter provide no more than 10 GL, while the snacks provide no more than 5 GL. Most are adapted from recipes in *The Low GL Diet Bible*, *The Low GL Diet Cookbook* or *Delicious, Healthy Sugar-Free*, all of which are packed with additional dishes. *The Low GL Diet Cookbook* is a good first step to increasing your repertoire of low GL recipes, while *Delicious, Healthy, Sugar-Free* includes slightly higher GL dishes that are great if you are entertaining (see Resources).

Breakfasts

Get Up & Go with CarboSlow®, Low Carb Milk and Berries (page 329)
Oat and Chia Porridge (page 329)
Yoghurt and Berries with Chopped Almonds (page 330)

Scrambled Eggs on Oatcakes or Pumpernickel (page 330)
Spiced Apples or Plums (page 330)
Low GL Granola (page 331)

Snacks

A piece of fruit plus 5 almonds or a dessertspoon of
pumpkin seeds
A thin piece of bread/2 oatcakes and half a small tub of cottage
cheese (150g/5¼oz)
A thin piece of bread/2 oatcakes and quarter of a small tub of
hummus (50g/1¾oz)
A thin piece of bread/2 oatcakes and peanut butter
Crudités (sliced carrot, pepper, cucumber or celery)
and hummus
Crudités and cottage cheese
A small, unsweetened, plain yoghurt (150g/5¼oz) and berries,
or soya berry yoghurt
Cottage cheese and berries
A slice of Low GL Carrot and Walnut Cake (page 331) or Apple
and Almond Cake (page 333)
Any of the snacks from the high fat phase (see Chapter 27)

Main Meals

Salads

A substantial serving of any of these provides 10 GLs. Or have half
a portion as a 5GL snack.

Apple and Tuna Salad (page 334)
Butternut Squash Salad (page 334)

Walnut and Three Bean Salad (page 335)
Salmon Stuffed Avocado (page 336)
Peruvian Quinoa Salad (page 336)
Olive, Pine Nut and Feta Salad (page 337)
Quinoa Tabbouleh (page 338)

Soups

Have a big bowl (300–350g/10½–16¼oz) of vegetable or bean soup.
Serve with two or three rough oatcakes.

Beany Vegetable Soup (page 339)
Chestnut and Butter Bean Soup (page 340)
Lentil and Lemon Soup (page 340)
Spicy Pumpkin and Tofu Soup (page 341)
High Energy Lentil Soup (page 342)
Summer Pea and Mint Soup (page 343)

Other Main Meals

Wholemeal Kamut Bulgur Pasta with Borlotti Bolognese
(page 344)
Kamut Bulgur Spaghetti with Chestnut Mushrooms and Truffle
Oil (page 345)
Thai Lamb Red Curry (page 346)
Chickpea and Spinach Curry (page 347)
Garlic Chilli Prawns with Pak Choi (page 348)
Sticky Mustard Salmon Fillets (page 349)
Trout with Puy Lentils and Roasted Tomatoes on the Vine
(page 350)

Recipes

Breakfasts

Get Up & Go with CarboSlow, Low Carb Milk and Berries

Add a teaspoon of chia seeds for extra protein, omega-3s and fibre. Make the shake watery, not too thick, and consume immediately after making. The glucomannan in CarboSlow absorbs liquid rapidly, and ideally this should happen inside you, as it will keep you feeling full for longer. Serves 1.

1 tbsp Get Up & Go with CarboSlow
480ml (17 fl oz) unsweetened soya or almond milk, or full fat cow's milk
Handful of blueberries, strawberries or raspberries

Blitz all of the ingredients in a blender.
8 GL/5g carbs

Oat and Chia Porridge

Half a chopped or stewed apple, plus some cinnamon, may be used instead of the berries, and/or chopped almonds, pecans or walnuts instead of the chia seeds. Add half a teaspoon of xylitol (0.5 GL) if required. Serves 1.

25g oats
120ml (4fl oz) carb free almond or soya milk
2 tsp chia seeds
Handful of berries

Simmer the oats in 240ml (8fl oz) of water and the milk for 5–10 minutes, then add the other ingredients.
10 GL/21g carbs

Yoghurt and Berries with Chopped Almonds

A satisfying, simple breakfast. Serves 1.

100g (3½oz) unsweetened sheep's, goat's, coconut or plain
soya yoghurt
Handful of blueberries, strawberries or raspberries
Small handful of chopped or flaked almonds

Fold the yoghurt and berries together, then sprinkle the
almonds on top.
5 GL/25g carbs

Scrambled Eggs on Oatcakes or Pumpernickel

If you want something a bit more substantial, a 25g (1oz) slice of
salmon may be added to the eggs. The eggs may be poached or
boiled (but not fried), rather than scrambled. Serves 1.

2 large eggs
2 or 3 rough oatcakes or a thin slice of pumpernickel

Scramble the eggs in a pan and add to the oatcakes/
punpernickel.
9 GL/14g carbs

Spiced Apples or Plums

A great, fruity start to the day. You can also use berries instead of
the apple/plums. Serves 1.

1 apple, chopped, or 4 plums, with the stones removed
A little water
Pinch of ground cinnamon to taste

2 tbsp Greek or coconut yoghurt
2–3 walnuts, chopped

Stew the apples/plums gently in the water until they soften.
Cool and serve with the yoghurt and a sprinkle of walnuts.
9 GL/20g carbs

Low GL Granola

A low GL granola that couldn't be easier. Serves 1.

60g (2oz) oats
60g (2oz) Lizi's Low GL Granola (available in UK supermarkets)
240ml (8fl oz) unsweetened oat, soya or full fat cow's milk
2 tsp chia or pumpkin seeds
Small handful of berries

Mix the oats and granola, pour over the milk and sprinkle over
the seeds and berries – simple and delicious.
5 GL/20g carbs

Snacks

Low GL Carrot and Walnut Cake

You can enjoy this fabulous teatime treat without feeling guilty.
The walnuts, carrots and eggs all help to lower the GL score and
provide plenty of nutrients. A slice is also delicious with a cup
of peppermint tea at the end of a long day. If you use the walnut
topping, the cake will keep well in an airtight tin for two days. If
you opt for the cream cheese frosting, cover the cake and store it
in the fridge. Again, it will keep for two days. You'll need a small
(10cm) cake tin to make this treat. Serves 4.

For the cake:

50g (1¾oz) coconut oil or butter (at room temperature), plus extra for greasing
50g (1¾oz) xylitol
50g (1¾oz) organic soya flour
¼ tsp baking powder
50g (1¾oz) walnuts, ground
50g (1¾oz) walnuts, chopped
1 medium carrot (75g/2¾oz), peeled and finely grated
2 medium eggs

For walnut topping:

2 tbsp chopped walnuts

For frosting:

50g (1¾oz) cream cheese
½ tsp vanilla extract
1 tsp xylitol

1 Preheat the oven to 180°C/350°F. Grease and line a 10cm (4in) cake tin with non-stick paper.
2 Cream the coconut oil or butter and xylitol together until soft and smooth.
3 Stir in the soya flour, baking powder and ground walnuts until the mixture resembles breadcrumbs.
4 Mix in the chopped walnuts and carrot, then stir in the eggs, without beating them.
5 Spoon into the prepared cake tin and sprinkle the chopped walnuts on top, if required. Bake for 35 minutes or until the top has risen and the colour is golden.
6 Remove from the oven and cover the top with foil, then bake for a further 20 minutes or until the cake is fully cooked. (Insert a skewer into the middle: if it comes out fairly clean,

then the cake is cooked; if the mixture is still runny, then it
needs a bit longer.)

7   To make the cream cheese frosting, if required, mix all
    of the ingredients together well. Allow the cake to cool
    thoroughly before spreading the frosting on top.

5 GL/12g carbs

Apple and Almond Cake

This recipe is a healthy take on Dorset apple cake (which is full of
butter and sugar). Our version provides all of the taste and texture
of the original, but without the gluten, sugar or dairy. It also provides plenty of fibre and minerals. It will keep well in an airtight
tin for up to two days. You will a small (10cm) cake tin. Serves 4.

50g (1¾oz) coconut oil or butter (at room temperature)
50g (1¾oz) xylitol
50g (1¾oz) organic soya flour
½ tsp baking powder
50g (1¾oz) ground almonds
50g (1¾oz) flaked almonds plus 1 tbsp for sprinkling on top
150g (5¼oz) unpeeled Bramley apples (cored weight), diced
2 medium eggs

1   Preheat the oven to 180ºC/350ºF. Grease and line a 10cm
    (4in) cake tin with non-stick paper. Alternatively, you
    could use two medium-sized muffin moulds, lined with
    paper liners.
2   Cream the coconut oil or butter and xylitol together until
    soft and smooth.
3   Stir in the flour, baking powder and ground almonds until
    the mixture resembles breadcrumbs.
4   Mix in the flaked almonds and apples, then stir in the eggs,
    without beating them.

5   Spoon into the cake tin and sprinkle the rest of the flaked almonds on top. Bake for 25 minutes or until the top is golden and set.

6   Remove from the oven and cover the top with a sheet of tin foil, then return to the oven for a further 20 minutes or until the cake is fully cooked. (Insert a skewer into the middle: if it comes out fairly clean, then the cake is cooked; if the mixture is still runny, then it needs a bit longer.)

5 GL/4g carbs

Main Meals

Apple and Tuna Salad

This is a refreshing salad when you want something simple, easy to prepare but a little different and satisfying. Serves 2.

175g (6oz) tin of tuna in brine, drained
1 apple, chopped
1 celery stick, sliced
1 little gem lettuce, torn into bite-sized pieces
1 tbsp mayonnaise
85g (3oz) plain yogurt
2 tsp lemon juice
Pinch of sea salt
Finely ground black pepper

Mix the tuna with the remaining ingredients.
6 GL/13g carbs

Butternut Squash Salad

This healthy salad can be served either warm or cold, ideally dressed with vinaigrette. Serves 3.

1 butternut squash, thinly sliced
A handful of broccoli florets or Tenderstem broccoli
300g (10½oz) bag of mixed salad leaves
6 sundried tomatoes, chopped
1 slice of halloumi cheese, diced
Vinaigrette to taste

1   Oven-bake the butternut squash at 180ºC/350ºF for 30
     minutes. Then peel and dice.
2   Steam the broccoli for 3 minutes.
3   Combine the oven-baked squash with the steamed broccoli,
     mixed salad leaves and the chopped sun-dried tomatoes.
4   Meanwhile, grill the halloumi cheese.
5   Add the cheese to the salad and dress the salad with
     vinaigrette. Serve warm or cold.
4 GL/8g carbs

Walnut and Three Bean Salad

This dish is so easy to prepare when you're pushed for time and
in need of a quick lunch or supper. Serves 2.

400g (14oz) can mixed beans, such as haricot beans, chickpeas
and flageolet beans
Handful of walnuts, roughly chopped
Half a small apple, cubed
2 tsp chopped fresh flat leaf parsley or chives
1 tbsp olive oil
1 tbsp walnut oil or olive oil
Juice of 1 lemon
1 celery stick, finely chopped
Pinch of sea salt
Freshly ground black pepper

Combine all of the ingredients and serve with the salad leaves.
3 GL/7g carbs

Salmon-Stuffed Avocado

A simple satisfying lunch. Serves 1.

1 avocado
3 tbsp smoked salmon pieces
1 tsp of lemon juice
Black pepper
Mixed green salad

1   Scoop the flesh from both halves of the avocado, and mash
    with the smoked salmon pieces, lemon juice and black
    pepper to taste.
2   Spoon back into the skins and serve with a mixed
    green salad.
1 GL/15g carbs

Peruvian Quinoa Salad

Quinoa is high in protein, as well as minerals. The inclusion of
pumpkin seeds further increases the mineral content. Serve with
green leaves or on its own. Serves 4

300g (10½oz) quinoa
Juice of up to 4 limes, or to taste, depending on how
juicy they are
1 good handful coriander leaves
2 good handfuls flat leaf parsley leaves
8 spring onions, finely sliced
1 clove garlic, crushed
4 tbsp pumpkin seeds

½ cucumber, finely diced
200g (7oz) cherry tomatoes, thinly sliced or diced
2 ripe avocadoes, diced (add these just before serving to prevent discolouration)
Good drizzle (around 4 tbsp) cold pressed, virgin rapeseed or olive oil
A little sea or rock salt
Freshly ground black pepper

1   Place the quinoa in a large saucepan, cover with double the volume of water and bring to the boil. Cover and simmer for around 12–13 minutes or until the water is absorbed and the grains are soft and fluffy.
2   Finely chop the fresh herbs and stir through the quinoa along with the rest of the ingredients except vinaigrette.
3   Taste to check the seasoning and add a little vinaigrette before serving if wished.

8 GL/15g carbs

Olive, Pine Nut and Feta Salad

Strong Mediterranean flavours and vivid colours make this a perfect summer lunch. It is a high scorer for antioxidants. It's perfect served with a simple green leaf salad. Serves 2

50g (2oz) Kalamata olives, halved
25g (1oz) sun-dried tomato pieces, chopped
75g (3oz) feta cheese, chopped or crumbled
2 tbsp pine nuts
2 tsp dried oregano
Juice of ¼ lemon
Freshly ground black pepper
2 small, ripe tomatoes, diced

100g (3½oz) mixed leaves, such as rocket, spinach and watercress

1   Mix the olives, sun-dried tomatoes, feta, pine nuts, oregano, lemon juice and pepper together in a bowl.
2   Stir in the fresh tomatoes, taste to check the flavour and adjust if necessary.
3   Serve over the salad leaves.

3 GL/5g carbs

Quinoa Tabbouleh

This uses quinoa in place of the traditional Kamut bulgur, as it is higher in protein and will keep you fuller for longer. Serves 2.

140g (5oz) quinoa
280ml (10fl oz) vegetable bouillon
Medium cucumber, sliced lengthways into quarters, then finely sliced horizontally
2 good handfuls of cherry tomatoes, chopped to the same size as the cucumber
4 spring onions, finely sliced
Large handful of fresh mint, finely chopped
Large handful of flat leaf parsley, finely chopped
1–2 tbsp olive oil
1 tbsp lemon juice
2 tsp balsamic vinegar (or to taste)
Pinch of sea salt
Finely ground black pepper

1   Bring the quinoa to the boil in a pan of water with the bouillon, then cover, reduce the heat and simmer for approximately 10–15 minutes, or until the liquid is fully absorbed and the grains are fluffy. Put the cooked quinoa in a bowl and leave to cool.

2　When the quinoa reaches room temperature, mix in the chopped vegetables and herbs, then add the oil, to taste, lemon juice and vinegar. Season to taste.

3　Place in the fridge for at least an hour to allow the flavours to develop.

8 GL/15g carbs

Beany Vegetable Soup

This simple soup takes just 30 minutes to prepare from start to finish. It is also full of fibre, so it will keep you feeling satisfied for longer. Serves 6.

2 onions, chopped
3 celery sticks, finely chopped
3 leeks, sliced
450g (1lb) mixed root vegetables, such as carrot, swede and parsnip, peeled and chopped into bite-sized chunks
850ml (34fl oz) vegetable stock
2 x 400g (14oz) cans mixed pulses (such as kidney, borlotti, butter or flageolet beans or chickpeas), drained and rinsed
2 tbsp roughly chopped flat leaf parsley
Pinch of sea salt
Freshly ground black pepper

1　Put the onion, celery, leeks, root vegetables, stock and seasoning in a large pan and stir.

2　Cover and bring to the boil, then reduce the heat and simmer for 20 minutes.

3　Stir in the mixed pulses, then cover and simmer for 5–10 minutes, or until the vegetables and pulses are tender.

4　Add the parsley and check the seasoning before serving.

8 GL/20g carbs

Chestnut and Butter Bean Soup

This is another easy soup to prepare when you feel in need of something light but comforting. You can use ready-cooked chestnuts (available in larger supermarkets) to save time and effort. Serves 4.

200g (7oz) cooked and peeled chestnuts (use vacuum-packed or canned to save time)
400g (14oz) can butter beans, drained and rinsed
1 onion, chopped
1 carrot, chopped
2 sprigs of thyme
1.2 litres (2½ pints) vegetable bouillon or stock
Freshly ground black pepper

1   Place all of the ingredients in a large pan and bring
    to the boil.
2   Cover and simmer very gently for 35 minutes. Remove
    the thyme.
3   Remove from the heat and purée in a blender until smooth.
4 GL/5g carbs

Lentil and Lemon Soup

The spices and lemony sharpness make this lentil soup anything but boring. It's a satisfying winter warmer. Serves 4.

1 tbsp olive oil
250g (9oz) onions, chopped
4 cloves of garlic, coarsely chopped
250g (9oz) red lentils, rinsed
1200ml (2½ pints) chicken or vegetable stock
1 tsp ground cumin

1 tsp ground coriander
Juice of ½ lemon
Pinch of sea salt
Freshly ground black pepper

1   Heat the oil in a pan, add the onions and garlic, and cook over
    a low heat, stirring frequently, for 10 minutes, or until soft.
2   Add the lentils and cook for a further 2 minutes.
3   Add the stock and bring to the boil, then reduce the heat to a
    simmer for 30–45 minutes, or until the lentils are almost soft.
4   In a non-stick frying pan, dry fry the spices over a high heat
    for 1–2 minutes, or until they release their aroma, then add
    to the soup.
5   Bring back to the boil, add the lemon juice, then simmer for
    5 minutes. Lightly season before serving.
2 GL/3g carbs

Spicy Pumpkin and Tofu Soup

This soup is full of flavour from the spices. It's worth taking the
time to dry fry them for a minute or two before you add the stock
in order to unlock their aroma. Serves 4.

1 tbsp olive oil
1 large onion, finely chopped
2 cloves of garlic, crushed
2 large butternut squashes, deseeded, peeled and diced
1½ tsp cumin
1 tsp ground coriander
¼ tsp chilli powder
½ tsp grated nutmeg
1 tsp fresh thyme, chopped
1.2 litre (2 pints) vegetable stock
1 packet Cauldron organic tofu, drained

Pinch of sea salt
Freshly ground black pepper
2 tbsp freshly chopped parsley and chives

1   Heat the olive oil in a large pan, then add the chopped onion
    and garlic, and gently cook over a low heat until the onion
    has softened.
2   Add the diced squash, cumin, coriander, chilli, nutmeg,
    thyme and stock, bring to the boil, then reduce the heat and
    simmer for 15 minutes before allowing to cool slightly.
3   Whizz the tofu in a food processor and set aside.
4   Blitz the soup in a blender and return to the pan, then whisk
    in the tofu, a tablespoon at a time.
5   Season to taste, add the fresh herbs, and serve.
Note: This recipe is courtesy of Cauldron Foods.
6 GL/15g carbs

High Energy Lentil Soup

This soup is packed with vitamin A from the carrots and tomatoes, as well as health-giving garlic. Serves 4.

2 tbsp olive oil
1 large onion, chopped
1 clove of garlic
2 sticks of celery, chopped
1 leek, sliced
1 carrot, sliced
200g (7oz) tin chopped tomatoes
1 tsp dried mixed herbs or 1 handful finely chopped parsley
200g (7oz) (dry weight) brown or green lentils
1 litre (2 pints) vegetable stock
Freshly ground black pepper

1   Heat the oil and a splash of water in a large lidded pan and

steam-fry the garlic, onion, celery and leek over a medium heat, turning frequently, until soft and transparent – about 8 minutes.

2   Add the remaining ingredients and stir thoroughly to combine. Bring to a simmer, then turn down the heat and add the lid.

3   Cook for 30–40 minutes or until the lentils and all the vegetables are tender.

4   Leave to cool slightly, then transfer half of the soup to a blender and blitz until smooth.

5   Return the blended soup to the pan, stir well to combine, reheat and serve.

4 GL/6g carb

Summer Pea and Mint Soup

This is our healthy take on a summer favourite. The recipe makes a large quantity of soup, which can be really useful if you want to prepare several meals in advance (for example, to take to work for lunch). For added flavour, crumbled goat's cheese or cubed rashers of lean bacon make a great topping. Serves 5.

1.5kg (3lb 5oz) frozen peas (or fresh peas, or half and half)
Leaves from 1 large bunch of fresh mint
Small tub crème fraîche
Salt and pepper, to taste

1   Bring a litre of water to the boil and add the peas and mint, reserving a few leaves for garnish. Return to the boil and simmer for 3 minutes.

2   Strain off most of the liquor but retain it, then blend the peas and mint until you have a smooth purée.

3   Add some of the liquor to the purée until you achieve the desired consistency.

4   Return to the pan and gently bring back to the boil. It is
    then cooked.
5   Season to taste. To serve, swirl a teaspoon of crème fraîche
    into each bowl of soup and add a mint leaf.

3 GL/5g carbs

Other Main Meals

Wholemeal Kamut Pasta with Borlotti Bolognese

If you can't get hold of Kamut pasta, there a number of high
fibre/high protein alternatives, such as black bean, green
lentil or chickpea pasta, all of which are now widely available.
Equally, you could use quinoa or spiralised ribbons of courgette. Serves 2.

1 tbsp olive oil
1 onion, chopped
2 cloves of garlic, crushed
1 tsp mixed dried herbs
115g (4oz) button mushrooms, sliced
1 tsp vegetable bouillon powder
1 tbsp tomato purée
140g (5oz) canned tomatoes
400g (14oz) can borlotti beans, drained and rinsed
Freshly ground black pepper
80g (3oz) wholemeal Kamut spaghetti or penne
Pinch of salt

1   Put the oil in a pan and sauté the onion, garlic and herbs for
    2 minutes, then add the mushrooms and cook until soft.
2   Add the vegetable bouillon powder, tomato purée, canned
    tomatoes and beans, season, then simmer for 15 minutes.
3   Meanwhile, bring a pan of water to the boil, add the pasta,

and simmer for about 8 minutes. Add a drop of olive oil to the water to stop the pasta sticking.

4   Drain the pasta when it is *al dente* and spoon the bolognese on top to serve.

10 GL/22g carbs

Kamut Spaghetti with Chestnut Mushrooms and Truffle Oil

Truffle oil is now quite easy to find, and it adds a massive amount of flavour to any dish. Serves 2.

1 tbsp ghee or butter
2 red onions, chopped
2 cloves of garlic, chopped
150g (5¼oz) chestnut mushrooms, sliced
1 dsp truffle oil
80g (3oz) Kamut spaghetti (or wholegrain spaghetti)
Freshly ground black pepper
2 tsp tahini

1   Sauté the onions and garlic in the ghee for 2 minutes, then add the mushrooms and continue to sauté for a further minute, stirring them so that they absorb the ghee and start to sweat. Add a dessertspoon of water if necessary, then the truffle oil.

2   Turn the heat down low and put a lid on the pan.

3   Meanwhile, bring a pan of water to the boil, add the Kamut pasta, and simmer for about 8 minutes. Add a drop of olive oil to the water to stop the pasta sticking.

4   Drain the pasta when it is *al dente* and stir into the mushroom mixture. Let it cook for a further minute, to enhance the flavour.

5   Add the black pepper and stir in the tahini.

6   Serve with a green salad, such as rocket and watercress with
    a drizzle of virgin olive oil and balsamic vinegar.
10 GL/18g carbs

Thai Lamb Red Curry

This warming curry is full of the flavours of Thailand. If you like a
bit of extra heat, you can always add some fresh red chillies. Serves 4.

1 tbsp coconut oil or virgin rapeseed oil
4 tsp Thai red curry paste
450g (1lb) lamb leg, diced
50g (2oz) unsalted cashew nuts, blitzed in a food processor
1 tbsp tomato purée
400ml (14fl oz) full fat coconut milk
2 lime leaves, roughly crumbled
200g (7oz) Kamut bulgur
150g (5¼oz) mangetout or fine green beans
1 tbsp fish sauce
Lime wedges, to serve

1   Heat the oil in a wok over a high heat.
2   Add the curry paste and stir fry for a minute, then add the
    lamb and stir fry to coat it in the paste.
3   Tip the cashew nuts, tomato purée, coconut milk and lime
    leaves into the wok and bring to the boil.
4   Reduce the heat slightly, cover and simmer, stirring
    occasionally, for around 50–60 minutes or until the sauce
    has reduced and thickened.
5   After about 45 minutes, bring a pan of water to the boil and
    cook the Kamut bulgur for 8 minutes.
6   Shortly before serving, boil or steam the mangetout or
    beans until *al dente*, then stir into the curry along with the
    fish sauce.

7   Serve with the Kamut bulgur and squeeze on the juice of the lime wedges.

8 GL/12g carbs

Chickpea and Spinach Curry

This no-frills curry is a terrific option when you're short of time. It makes use of mixed spices and pre-cooked chickpeas. Serves 4.

1 tbsp olive oil or coconut oil
2 red onions, sliced
1 mild red chilli, deseeded and finely chopped
1 tbsp mild or medium curry powder (or Madras spice blend)
150ml (⅓ pint) vegetable stock
500ml (1 pint) coconut milk
¼ of a cauliflower, chopped into smallish chunks
2 x 410g (14¼oz) cans chickpeas, rinsed and drained
200g (7oz) baby leaf spinach, chopped
200g (7oz) Kamut bulgur or 160g (5½oz) quinoa
1 tsp sea salt

1   Heat half of the oil in a large pan, add the onions, and cook for 3–4 minutes to soften.
2   Add the chilli and curry powder and cook for a further minute.
3   Stir in the stock, coconut milk, cauliflower pieces and chickpeas, then simmer for 15 minutes to reduce the sauce and allow the flavours to combine. Season with salt.
4   Meanwhile, bring a pan of water to the boil and cook the Kamut bulgur for 8 minutes (or the quinoa for 10–15 minutes).
5   A couple of minutes before you want to serve, stir the spinach into the curry and let it warm through.

6   Serve with the Kamut bulgur (or quinoa).
10 GL/15g carbs

Note: A salad of diced cucumber, tomatoes and red onion is a
good accompaniment.

Garlic Chilli Prawns with Pak Choi

A simple marinade adds a lot of flavour to the prawns to make
this a tasty and satisfying meal. You can simply add chilli flakes
to normal oil if you are unable to find chilli infused oil. Serves 2.

For the marinated prawns:
3 cloves of garlic, crushed
Juice of 2 limes
1 green chilli, de-seeded
1 tbsp chilli infused oil (or dried chilli flakes in normal oil)
Large pinch of sea salt
3 tbsp virgin rapeseed oil
300g (10½oz) large fresh, raw prawns, fully prepared

For the vegetables:
1 tbsp virgin rapeseed oil
250g (9oz) pak choi, stems separated from the leaves, and both
stems and leaves roughly chopped
Oyster sauce

For accompaniment:
100g (3½oz) Kamut bulgur or 80g (2¾oz) quinoa (dry weight)

1   Blend the garlic, lime, chilli, chilli oil, salt and oil to purée.
2   Use this mixture to marinate the prawns for 20 minutes at
    room temperature.

3 Bring a pan of water to the boil and cook the Kamut bulgur for 8 minutes (or the quinoa for 10–15 minutes).

4 Cook the prawns for 1½ minutes per side in a medium hot griddle pan or frying pan.

5 Add the rapeseed oil to a hot wok or frying pan and stir fry or steam fry the pak choi for around 4 minutes, adding the stems to the pan first to cook for a minute before you add the leaves.

6 Once cooked, remove from the heat and stir through the oyster sauce to taste.

7 Serve immediately with the prawns and the Kamut bulgur (or quinoa).

10 GL/18g carbs

Sticky Mustard Salmon Fillets

This dish requires a bit of planning as you need to allow enough time to marinate the fillets before cooking. However, thereafter, they are simply baked, which gives you plenty of time to prepare everything else, so this is a great option when you have people over for dinner. Serves 2.

Juice and grated rind of ½ an orange
1 tsp clear honey
1 tsp wholegrain mustard
2 small skinless, boneless salmon fillets
Large bunch of spinach
1 or 2 red or yellow peppers, chopped
100g (3½oz) Kamut bulgur or 80g (2¾oz) quinoa, or 3 baby new potatoes, boiled

1 Whisk the orange juice and rind into the mustard and honey.

2 Place the salmon fillets in a shallow dish and pour over the

orange mixture. Leave to marinate for 30–60 minutes in the fridge.

3   Preheat the oven to 180°C/350°F then bake the salmon for 20–25 minutes.

4   Meanwhile, bring a pan of water to the boil and cook the Kamut bulgur, quinoa or new potatoes.

5   Five minutes before serving, steam fry the spinach and red or yellow peppers.

10 GL/17g carbs

Trout with Puy Lentils and Roasted Tomatoes on the Vine

Lentils are a great low GL and filling alternative to grains, and they go fantastically well with fish. This is a really flavourful dish. Serves 2.

85g (3oz) (dry weight) Puy lentils, washed and drained
1 tsp vegetable bouillon powder
1 tsp mixed dried herbs
2 small trout fillets
12 cherry tomatoes on the vine
2 slices of lemon
Handful of fresh flat leaf parsley, chopped
Finely ground black pepper

1   Cover the lentils with cold water and bring to the boil, then simmer for about 20 minutes, or until the water has been more or less absorbed.

2   Add the bouillon powder and mixed herbs when the lentils are soft to the bite. (Don't worry if they seem a little hard – Puy lentils retain their shape and have a satisfyingly chewy texture when cooked.)

3   Place the fish in a non-stick roasting tin and lay the

tomatoes around them, then bake at 190°C/375°F for 12–15 minutes or until cooked through.

4   Put a dollop of lentils onto each plate and lay the fillets on top.

5   Add a slice of lemon and chopped parsley to each fillet, then put the cooked tomatoes on the side. Sprinkle with black pepper.

10 GL/14g carbs

Chapter 29

What to Drink

The best drink for both general health and fat burning is water. You should aim to consume the equivalent of 2 litres (4 pints) – or eight glasses – each day. If this seems an enormous amount, bear in mind that you can factor in tea and coffee (and the occasional juice in the slow carb phase).

Leaving a bottle of water on your desk will remind you to keep it topped up. Like the rest of the Hybrid Diet, drinking plenty of fluid will eventually become second nature. And it will leave you feeling much better in every way.

Cold Drinks and Juices

You must avoid fruit juice during the high fat phase. Actually, this is a pretty good principle to follow at all times, although a half-shot of Blueberry Active (made from pure blueberries) or Cherry Active (made from Montmorency cherries) is low GL and very high in antioxidants, so it might be worth working out a way to include it in the slow carb phase.

All commercial fruit juices, whether concentrated or freshly squeezed, have a relatively high GL because the fibre has been removed. The best is probably cloudy apple juice, although even this should be drunk diluted – half juice/half water or, even better, two-thirds water/one-third juice.

The following table indicates 5 GL portions for a variety of drinks. Remember, you have a daily 5 GL allowance in the slow carb phase for drinks or desserts.

Drink	Serving size
Tomato juice	500ml (approx.1 pint)
Carrot juice	Small glass
Grapefruit juice, unsweetened	Small glass
Apple juice, unsweetened	Small glass, diluted 50/50 with water
Orange juice, unsweetened	Small glass, diluted 50/50 with water; or freshly squeezed juice of 1 orange
Blueberry Active	20ml (1 tbsp) of concentrate
Cherry Active	20ml (1 tbsp) of concentrate
Pineapple juice	Half a small glass, diluted 50/50 with water
Cranberry juice	Half a small glass, diluted 50/50 with water
Grape juice	2cm (1in) in a glass – avoid!

Stay away from all fizzy, sweetened and caffeinated drinks as well as sugar-sweetened cordials.

A good rule of thumb is to have no more than one glass of juice each day, diluting it as need be so that you never have more than 5 GLs in the course of the day. So, you could have either a small glass of carrot juice or a small glass of diluted apple juice – not both!

Always drink slowly – sip rather than gulp – as this helps to retard the release of the sugars in the juice (as does diluting).

Coffee, Tea and Chocolate

It may be a good idea to have a coffee with full fat cream or coconut oil first thing in the morning during the high fat phase. In addition to acting as an energiser and appetite suppressant, this will increase ketone levels and encourage the body to release stored fat, which the liver can then convert into more ketones. One recent study gave a group of volunteers the equivalent of either two or four cups of coffee and found that the higher dose had a greater impact on level of ketones.[1] Another trial found that MCT oil also raises ketones,[2] so the coffee–coconut oil combination should be pretty effective. C8 oil would be even better, although we recommend drinking this as a shot, as it would just float on the top of the coffee.

A 2014 study also concluded that coffee drinkers have less risk of developing diabetes than non-coffee drinkers.[3] On the other hand, two years later, a meta-analysis of seven previous trials asserted that caffeine makes the body less sensitive to insulin, which causes blood sugar to rise: 'Acute caffeine ingestion reduces insulin sensitivity in healthy subjects. Thus, in the short term, caffeine might shift glycemic homeostasis toward hyperglycemia,' reported the authors.[4] If true, this would be bad news for coffee addicts. On a personal level, I (Patrick) have found that drinking straight coffee (not in a Hybrid Latté) tends to raise my blood sugar by about 1mmol/l for an hour or so.

Another study also found that insulin sensitivity deteriorates and blood sugar level rises as caffeine dose increases.[5] This suggests that it is something else in coffee – not the caffeine – that provides protection against diabetes, especially as decaf has no impact on insulin sensitivity. Then again, the explanation for this apparent paradox – coffee drinkers are less susceptible to diabetes yet caffeine reduces insulin sensitivity – may be quite straightforward. As coffee is an effective appetite suppressant, coffee drinkers may simply eat fewer carbs than non-coffee drinkers, which would reduce their risk of developing diabetes over the long term. Some people gravitate towards sugar for an instant energy boost, whereas others prefer coffee. The latter also has the benefit of a hit of antioxidants in every cup, especially if they drink filter coffee. (Some of the caffeine is filtered out, but none of the antioxidants.)

One thing is certain: coffee is much more harmful when it is drunk with a high carb snack. A group of researchers gave volunteers a carbohydrate snack, such as a croissant, muffin or toast, together with either decaf or caffeinated coffee.[6] Those in the second group experienced far greater increases in blood sugar (on average, their levels rose three times more than those who drank decaf), and their insulin sensitivity almost halved. So, drinking coffee with carbs should be avoided at all times.

The jury is still out on whether caffeine is bad for the heart. Numerous trials and studies have reported conflicting results, which may be due to the fact that about 40 per cent of people are fast caffeine metabolisers – that is, they experience a rapid but short-lived effect – whereas about 15 per cent are slow caffeine metabolisers who get a more gradual but longer boost. Both of these tendencies are inherited and cannot be changed. The latter group have an increased risk of both heart disease[7] and high blood pressure.[8]

There are a few more points to consider, too. For instance, coffee can increase the level of the amino acid homocysteine by as much as 11 per cent in under four hours.[9] Homocysteine is the best indicator of faulty methylation, which can result in many serious health problems, most notably memory loss and Alzheimer's disease. Coffee also inhibits sirtuin genes,[10] while both green tea and cacao/cocoa are sirtuin activators (see Chapter 20). Active sirtuin genes play a key role in fat burning and muscle growth and retention, so you certainly don't want to inhibit them.

If you love your coffee, our advice is to have one in the morning, without any food, and monitor your glucose and ketone levels (see Chapter 26). You should certainly avoid it after midday because it suppresses melatonin (which you need to sleep well) for up to ten hours. So, you could include coffee in a Hybrid Latté every morning, but try to resist the temptation to have another after lunch.

Green and Black Tea

From every point of view, we recommend green tea rather than black tea, although the latter is not bad either. For instance, green tea lowers blood glucose and improves insulin sensitivity, according to a meta-analysis of seventeen trials.[11] However, it has neither a positive nor a negative effect on diabetics.[12] Tea also contains theanine, a relaxing amino acid that counters the adrenalising impact of the caffeine it contains. Traditionally, the Japanese left green tea leaves in the pot and used them to make a run-through if they wanted another drink. Such run-throughs have relatively more antioxidants and polyphenols and relatively less caffeine.

Cacao, the sirtuin activator in dark chocolate, also helps to improve insulin sensitivity[13] and lower blood sugar. Dark chocolate is also an appetite suppressant (in marked contrast to either white or milk chocolate), so it's by far the best option as long as you eat a low GL variety.[14] In practical terms, this means it needs to be 80 per cent cacao. If you use sugar-free cacao powder and low GL milk (such as unsweetened soya or carb free almond milk) to make hot chocolate, you can always sweeten it with a little xylitol. Note that we also include a teaspoon of unsweetened raw cacao powder in our Hybrid Latté.

Alcohol

Pure alcohol, such as a neat shot of vodka, tequila, gin or whisky, has 0 GL and can even raise ketones. However, inevitably, it's not all good news!

First, even pure alcohol contains calories that your body will burn in preference to fat. Moreover, the liver can convert any alcohol that is not burned for energy directly into triglycerides, which can then be converted into ketones (which is why you sometimes see an increase in ketones after drinking). However, if you are not in ketosis, this increase in triglycerides will just make you fat. This is why alcohol consumption is routinely associated with weight gain. On the other hand, if you are in ketosis and drink too much alcohol, the body will be able to meet all its energy requirements from the booze and will stop converting body fat into ketones. So, go easy.

Second, alcohol is a toxin, so the body has to flush it out of the system, which interferes with normal, healthy metabolism. Third, it contains no nutrients. Finally, and perhaps most importantly, it weakens willpower, which might leave you scoffing carbs in the evening despite your best intentions.

It will take less alcohol than usual to leave you feeling drunk during ketosis, so, for this reason alone, it's a good idea to limit yourself to a maximum of one drink per day in the high fat phase. Moreover, if you drink any more than this, you are likely to suffer a very bad hangover.

Hangovers are due to a combination of dehydration and the generation of a toxin called acetaldehyde in the liver. So, to counteract the first, make sure you drink a large glass of water with every alcoholic drink. As for the acetaldehyde, one study gave a group of volunteers alcohol followed by either mineral water or a modest dose of theracurmin, a water-soluble form of curcumin (a compound that is found in turmeric). The level of acetaldehyde was cut by about a third in the second group.[15] We recommend both – curcumin and plenty of water – both during and after drinking alcohol. What's more, a recent trial found that curcumin protects the liver and reduces the risk of fatty liver disease.[16]

During both the high fat and slow carb phases, it's advisable to stick to those drinks that have the least carbs. So, dry white wine – or champagne – is better than dessert wine. Remember, during the slow carb phase, you have a daily allowance of 5 GLs for all drinks and desserts. So, assuming you've had no fruit juice or desserts during the day, you can allow yourself up to 5 GLs of alcohol.

As you will see from the table below, from a GL standpoint, your best options are neat spirits, then white wine, red wine and finally beer. If you are a beer drinker, you should limit yourself to just half a pint every other day (or choose a low carb beer). By contrast, if you prefer dry white wine, you can have a glass every day and still have 4 GLs left over for a dessert or a small glass of diluted apple juice.

Drink	GL	Units	Daily Maximum
Beer/lager ½ pint	10	1	¼ pint
Red wine small glass (115ml)	2	1	1
White wine small glass (115ml)	1	1	1
Spirit shot (30 ml)	0	1	1
Spirit and orange juice (125ml juice)	6	1	1 small
Spirit and Coke (125ml Coke)	8	1	1 very small

Note: We advise a daily maximum of no more than 5 GLs or 1 unit.

Finally, remember that the Ketonix breathalyser can give false readings after drinking alcohol, so do not measure you ketones in this way until at least twelve hours have passed since your last drink.

References and Further Sources of Information

Hundreds of highly respected scientific studies were consulted during the research for this book. Full details of – and links to – these reports are available at: www.hybriddiet.co.uk/references.

Recommended Reading

Nina Teicholtz, *The Big Fat Surprise: Why Butter, Meat and Cheese Belong in a Healthy Diet,* Simon & Schuster (2014)

Miriam Kalamian, *Keto for Cancer: Ketogenic Metabolic Therapy as a Targeted Nutritional Strategy,* Chelsea Green (2017)

Travis Christofferson and Dominic D'Agostino (Foreword), *Tripping Over the Truth: How the Metabolic Theory of Cancer is Overturning One of Medicine's Most Entrenched Paradigms,* Chelsea Green (2017)

Patrick Holford, *Say No To Cancer,* Piatkus 2010

Mary T. Newport, *Alzheimer's Disease: What if there was a cure and nobody knew?,* Basic Health Publications (2011)

Patrick Holford, *The Alzheimer's Prevention Plan,* Piatkus (2011)

Joesph R. Kraft, *Diabetes Epidemic & You,* Trafford Publishing (2008)

Patrick Holford, *Say No to Diabetes,* Piatkus (2011)

Malcolm Kendrick, *The Great Cholesterol Con*, John Blake Publishing (2008)

Patrick Holford, *Say No to Heart Disease*, Piatkus (2010)

Patrick Holford *The Low-GL Diet Bible*, Piatkus (2009)

Cookbooks

Patrick Holford and Fiona McDonald Joyce, *The Low-GL Diet Cookbook*, Piatkus (2005)

Patrick Holford and Fiona McDonald Joyce, *Delicious, Health, Sugar-Free*, Piatkus (2017)

Patrick Holford and Fiona McDonald Joyce, *The 10 Secrets of 100% Health Cookbook*, Piatkus (2012)

Jimmy Moore and Maria Emmerich, *The Ketogenic Cookbook*, Victory Belt Publishing (2015)

Recommended Viewing

Dr Thomas Dayspring's analysis of heart risk data is discussed in this interview (at 2 minutes and 42 seconds): https://thefatnurse. wordpress.com/2012/05/19/hdl-not-useful-anymore-maybe-the-whole-lipid-profile-is-useless/

Resources

General Information

Hybriddiet.co.uk

The website www.hybriddiet.co.uk provides support material for this book. You'll also find information on our worldwide seminars, webinar and retreats, plus products and services that can support you on the Hybrid Diet.

100% Health Check

You can have your own personal health and nutrition assessment online using Patrick Holford's 100% Health Check. This gives you a personalised assessment of your current health, and what you most need to change, including a metabolic check to gauge your risk of metabolic syndrome, and a BioAge Check. Visit www.patrickholford.com and go to 'FREE health check'.

100% Health Club

If you join the 100% Health Club you'll get a 40-page report after completing the 100% Health Check, and unlimited access to address your needs as your health improves. You also receive Patrick Holford's 100% Health newsletter every other month, plus instant access to all past newsletters online; special reports each month, to keep you motivated and informed (and access to his library of hundreds of reports on important health issues); a hotline to use via the private 100% Health members Facebook group; 20% off most seminars and events; up to 30% off all books and supplements from HOLFORDirect.com (up to 15% on foods); and a free copy of a Patrick Holford book on joining. Membership costs £7.99 a month.

The Brain Bio Centre
The Brain Bio Centre is an outpatient clinic of the charitable Food for the Brain Foundation in London, which specialises in the nutritional treatment of mental health issues, ranging from depression and insomnia to Alzheimer's and Parkinson's disease, under the direction of Patrick Holford. The Centre's team of expert nutritional therapists, backed up by a psychiatrist and neurologist, work with you to identify any nutritional and biochemical imbalances that may be contributing to your symptoms, and the consultation provides you with a tailored programme to correct these issues and restore your health. Through a process of nutritional and psychiatric assessment, appropriate clinical tests, dietary advice and supplements will then be recommended. Visit www.brainbiocentre.com or tel: +44 (0) 20 8332 9600.

The Food for the Brain Foundation
The Food for the Brain Foundation is a non-profit educational charity, founded by Patrick Holford, which aims to promote awareness of the link between learning, behaviour, mental health and nutrition; and to educate and provide educational material to children, parents, teachers, schools, the public, the catering industry, health professionals and the government. The website has a free Cognitive Function Test. It takes 15 minutes to complete. Depending on your score, it tells you what to do to improve your memory. For more information visit www.foodforthebrain.org.

Institute for Optimum Nutrition

The Institute for Optimum Nutrition (ION), founded by Patrick Holford, offers a three-year diploma course in nutritional therapy. Visit www.ion.ac.uk, address: Ambassador House, Paradise Rd, Richmond TW9 1SQ 2JY, UK, tel.: +44 (0)20 8614 7815.

Find a Nutritional Therapist

BANT, the British Association of Nutrition and Lifestyle Medicine, is the official register of qualified nutritional therapists. You can search for a therapist by area and see their specialisms should you need support with your health issues. See www.bant.org.uk.

We train nutritional therapists to support clients, so it is worth asking them if they are up to speed on the Hybrid Diet.

In Ireland see the Nutritional Therapist of Ireland at www.ntoi.ie.

Supplements

Patrick Holford has formulated a range of supplements to support optimal health. The backbone of a supplement programme is an optimum multivitamin and mineral, with extra vitamin C and essential fats, both omega-3 and 6. These are provided in the Optimum Nutrition Pack. If you are over 50, the enhanced version, the 100% Health Pack, provides extra anti-oxidants, including all the nutrients to support the Hybrid Diet – except carnitine, HCA and high dose chromium.

Cinnachrome® provides Cinnulin®, a potent extract of cinnamon, with 200mcg of chromium which contributes to normal nutrient metabolism and to the maintenance of normal blood glucose levels.

Carboslow® is a source of super-soluble glucomannan fibre, a highly soluble plant fibre that fills the stomach to give a feeling of satiety. Glucomannan contributes to weight loss as part of a calorie restricted diet. This effect is obtained with a daily intake of 3g glucomannan in three doses of 1g each, together with 1–2 glasses of water before meals. Glucomannan also contributes to the maintenance of normal blood cholesterol levels with a daily intake of 4 grams. In the US and Canada, PGX® is the leading super-soluble fibre that supports weight loss, blood sugar control and satiation.

Get Up & Go®

Get Up & Go is a delicious breakfast shake which is a combination of vitamins, minerals, essential fats, protein and fibre, and designed to be mixed into a tasty shake. One serving is just 8 GLs and is perfect for those following a low GL, slow carb diet.

There is no need to take a multivitamin and mineral if you have Get Up & Go since it provides optimal level of all vitamins and minerals.

Get Up & Go with Carboslow® provides 1 gram of glucomannan with each serving – see above. Served with carb-free milk (such as almond) and a small handful of berries, it is only approximately 5 GLs, hence it is suitable in both the high fat and slow carb phase.

GL Support is a combination of Garcinia Cambogia, 5-HTP and chromium. There is a version with carnitine.

GL Support may be particularly useful for those following a diet or exercise plan. Chromium contributes to normal nutrient metabolism and to the maintenance of normal blood glucose levels. Garcinia Cambogia, a natural source of HCA, may contribute to weight management and healthy appetite control. GL Support also contains B vitamins that help energy metabolism and contribute to a reduction in tiredness and fatigue, including vitamin B6 which contributes to normal protein and glycogen metabolism.

Hybrid Pack combines all the support nutrients you need in either a high fat or slow carb phase for optimal metabolic efficiency.

Ketofast® is a pure form of C8 oil, the most effective MCT oil. Each tablespoon provides 15ml of pure C8 derived from coconut oil, without any additives. Each bottle provides 30 x 15ml servings.

Mood and Awake Food provides 5-HTP and Tyrosine, and adaptogenic herbs to support recovery from addiction.

All Patrick Holford products are available from good health food shops and direct from www.HOLFORDirect.com or call 0370 3341575.

Other reputable supplement suppliers include:
Biocare – see www.biocare.co.uk
Solgar – see www.solgar-vitamins.co.uk
Higher Nature – see www.highernature.co.uk
Viridian – see www.viridian-nutrition.com.

Foods
Kamut khorosan This ancient form of wheat is becoming more widely available in many organic and health food shops and bakeries in Europe. In the UK, Doves Farm Foods sells Organic Kamut khorasan wholemeal flour online: www.dovesfarm.com Kamut pasta and bulgur is available from www.HOLFORDirect.com. Visit www.kamut.com, and select your country, to see a full list of what is available.

Longo's Five Day Package, to support his Fasting Mimicking Diet, contains plant-based energy bars, soups and a variety of snacks, and is available from https://prolonfmd.com/5.

Exogenous Ketone Supplements

There are three forms of exogenous ketones: C8 oil (see Ketofast above), which has to be converted in the liver into ketones; ketone salts such as KetoCaNa, currently only available in the US; and ketone esters, also available in the US from www.hvmn.com. Ketone esters are currently held up with a 'novel foods application' in the EU. We hope that they will shortly become available in the UK and the rest of the EU.

Glucose and Ketone Testing

Ketosticks measure ketone levels in urine. They are available from pharmacies or online and are relatively inexpensive. They are a basic way of knowning if you're in ketosis but they're not nearly as accurate as blood or breath testing.

Ketonix® breath analyser is the easiest and one of the cheaper ways of measuring ketones because you buy the device and can then use it as often as you wish – and anyone else can also use it. The tubular device has two parts – the device and a battery part that you charge up then attach so that you can use it away from a power source. Alternatively, you can connect it directly to your computer through a USB port. Normally, it costs around £168 but, at the time of writing, if you use the code HYBRID you will get 10% off (price is set in dollars). Go to www.ketonix. com/hybrid.

KEYA® Smart is a simple to use but state of the art monitor for testing glucose and ketones at the same time from a pin prick of blood that is fed onto a strip inserted into the monitor. It then records and shows you your ketone and glucose level and records all results so that you can see your trends as you try different phases of the hybrid diet. The best deal is to get the 'KEYA® Smart Meter Kit + 3 vials' which gives you 110 test strips each providing a combined glucose–ketone test. That's enough for a month's worth of testing, three times a day. The pack includes the premium colour touchscreen meter, lancing device, 25 lancets, micro-USB cable, wall charger, carry case, control solution, quick start guide and instruction booklet. At the time of writing it costs £189. It is easy to use and the instruction booklet explains everything very clearly. Go to www.keyasmart.com. The cost of strips, when you need more, works out much cheaper than monitors that require different strips for glucose and ketones.

Freestyle Libre is a glucose monitoring system designed to liberate patients from the hassles of glucose monitoring by attaching a sensor to your arm. This is painless. By placing the monitor near to your arm you can read your glucose level at any time. At the time of writing, the reader costs £58 and so does the sensor. Sensors last for two weeks only. Freestyle Libre is registered for use by diabetics only. For more details visit https://www.freestylelibre.co.uk.

Other Tests

HbA1c, homocysteine and IgG food intolerances: YorkTest (www.yorktest.com) offer HbA1c (glycosylated haemoglobin – the best measure of your blood sugar status) home-to-laboratory testing from a finger prick of blood, as part of an overall health testing package. They also have a self-test kit for measuring your homocysteine level and for identifying food intolerances, called Food Scan. The FoodScan 113 identifies the foods causing the intolerance and the level of intolerance. In addition, the service includes nutritionist consultations and comprehensive support and advice on managing your elimination diet. To order call YorkTest Laboratories on 0800 130 0580 or visit www.yorktest.com.

Insulin testing: Your GP is unlikely to sanction it on the NHS for heart disease but online test kits are available from www.medichecks.com/diabetes-tests/insulin-resistance-test for around

£50. You can combine the result with that from a fasting glucose test (more easily obtainable) in an online 'Homa' calculator to work out your level of insulin resistance. For more information on this see: https://www.diabetes.co.uk/forum/threads/insulin -testing-which-tests-on-the-nhs.128969/. This link shows you what your levels mean if you have them tested, based on Dr Kraft's research – www.meridianvalleylab.com/kraft-prediabetes-profil e-patterns-overview/.

Index

A

acetoacetate (AcAc) 48, 189, 286, 288–9
aceylation stimulating protein (ASP) 93, 129
addiction, and ketogenic and slow carbs 151–2
ADHD 110–11, 162
Agricultural Revolution 163, 165–6
alpha linolenic acid (ALA) 261
Alzheimer's:
    and brain disease? 51–2
    and coconut 50
    and glucose deficiency 50–2
    and mTOR 113
Alzheimer's Disease (Newport) 49
Alzheimer's Research 49, 54
American Institute of Cancer 211
American National Institutes of Health 50
anger through sugar 113–14
anti-addiction actions 156–7
approach for all cancers, ketogenic diet for 32–3 (*see also* cancer cells)
Argentina 80
Aricept 55
Atkins diet 43, 169
ATP 120–1
    as main energy 29–30
Australia 10
Australian Health Practitioners' Regulatory Authority 10
autophagy, switching on 126, 132–6, 208
    working of 133
Avena, Nicole 151
avoiding starchy veg 200–1
Avon Longitudinal Study 169

B

Babylonians 168
Banting, William 43
Bantu 167
Bariatric Medical Clinic 153
beta-glucuronidase, 107
beta-hydroxybutyrate (BHB) 48, 189, 286, 288, 289–90
Big Fat Surprise (Teicholz) 5, 11–12

biotin 48
Bissell, Mina 108–9
blood glucose level, ideal 292–3
Blum, Kenneth 153
BMJ 8
body mass index (BMI) 80
Boston University 24
bowel cancer, *see* colorectal
    cancer
brain:
    addicted, illustrated 148
    fruit and veg good for 194
    reclaiming 152–5
Brain Bio Centre 110–11
brain cancer (*see also* cancer and
    high carbs; monitoring diet):
    and Alzheimer's? 51–2
    and Charles's story 26–7, 28
    common side effects of 26
    and Raffi's story 23–4
Brand-Miller, Jenny 163
breast cancer:
    and blood-sugar level 106
    and GL diets 108
    one of top five 105
    rises in 105
    and women with high insulin
        levels 108
Bredesen, Dale 55
Bristol University 213
British Journal of Psychiatry
    113–14
British Medical Journal 12, 91–2
Brookhaven National Laboratory
    150
butyric acid 107

C

Canada 81–2, 88
cancer cells:
    and healthy cells 29
    and little to generate energy
        30
    voracious for sugar 23
cancer and dairy products 213–14
Cancer Genome Atlas 28–9
cancer and high carbs 104–9, 211
    (*see also* brain cancer)
    changing diet to reduce risk
        106–8
    inexorable rise of 104–5
Cancer Research Fund 106
Cancer Research UK 109
'carb fast' 219
carbohydrate, different types of
    17
'Carbohydrate–Insulin Model of
    Obesity' 44–5, 122
CarboSlow 239
cardio and strength training 144
cardiovascular health:
    evidence 97–100
    and strength training 144–5
carnitine: essential in high fat
    phase 276–7
Caucasian 212
C8 48
Center for Science in the Public
    Interest 12
changing diet to reduce risk
    106–8
Charing Cross Hospital 27
Cheraskin, Emanuel 272
Chestnut and Butter Bean Soup
    266

chia, with highest concentration 183

Children's Hospital, Boston 45, 91, 151

chimpanzees 159

China 80, 83, 93, 99, 107, 161, 167, 201

cholesterol (*see also* high-fat, low-carb):
blaming carbs, instead of 95–6
made in liver 9
myth 36–7

Cholesterol Treatment Trialists Collaboration organisation 36–7

Christofferson, Travis 28–9

chromium polynicotinate 281

chromium reverses insulin resistance 280–1

chylomicrons 9

Clarke, Kieran 50, 53

co-enzyme Q (Co-Q) 274–6, 283

Coca-Cola 7–8

cocaine 149, 153, 154

Coconut Collective 231

coconut oil, miracle of 52–5

Cognitive Function Test 115

cognitive function test 114–15

colorectal cancer:
and high GL diets 107
one of top five 105, 174
second most prevalent 210–13

Columbia University 111

Comprehensive Digestive Stool Analysis 213

cow's milk, two types of 166

Crawford, Michael 160, 162, 169

Credit Suisse 8

Cross, Helen 56

Crowe, Ivan 165

CTT, *see* Cholesterol Treatment Trialists Collaboration organisation

Cummings, Ivor 39

Cunnane, Stephen 50, 51–2, 53, 55, 162

Cutler, Richard 193

cytokines 20

D

dairy, not the answer 130–1

dairy products and cancer products 213–14

Dayspring, Thomas 37

dementia:
and developing, among adolescents 112–13
and diabetes 111
and ketones 50, 54
two-thirds of all cases 112

Department of Psychiatry, Oxford 154

diabetes (*see also* Unwin, David):
blood sugar stabilises 281
and drugs to combat 15–16
high GL equals high risk of 79–83
impressive trials for patients of 20
and insulin resistance 281
and kidneys 205
and low GL 75–6
and non-diabetics 49
and prediction by 2015 74
and protein, too much 208
UK diagnosis 15
Unwin treats for 16

diabetes – *continued*
and weight loss 16
   Wendy, example 85–6
   worldwide effect of 15
diabetes.co.uk 16, 18–19
Diabetes UK 16–17
  and low evidence for 'long-
    term safety' 17
'Dietary Guidelines for
   Americans' 5, 11–12
Dietitians Association of
   Australia 10
dopamine:
  and different proteins 205
  release of 148
dual fuel, becomes a problem
   127–8
dual fuel system and
   evolutionary advantage 171–2
Dubai 112–13

E

eating badly equals 'eatwell'
   12–14
eating more/less 267–8
'Eatwell Guide' 12–14, 74
Ebbeling, Cara 91
elemental energy 279–80
Elliott, Jennifer 10
energy, supplements for 281–2
enzymes (*see also*
   micronutrients, as hybrid
   support):
  and different proteins 205
  and mTOR 142
EPICOR 98
epilepsy, and counteract of
   ketogenic 55

evolution in hybrid sense 158–82
  and *Homo aquaticus* 159–62
  neural connections per second
    158–9
evolutionary advantage and dual
   fuel system 171–2

F

Facebook 148
Fasting-Mimicking Diet 140–2
fat, in chylomicrons 9
fat cholesterol con 9–12
fat-storing hormones, foods that
   trigger 128–30
fats, good 181–92
  for fuel 185–6
  and going nuts 187
  good, to eat 190–2
  illustrated 218
  intake of 217–18
  and MCT oil and synthetic
    ketones 189–90
  meat- and dairy-free phase 231
  most anti-inflammatory 183
  trans, avoiding 187–9
Feltham, Sam 3–4
Fettke, Gary 10, 11
Finland 114
Fishkins 204
5-HTP 156, 157, 281, 282, 364
Food for the Brain Foundation
   110–11
food diversity, loss of 167–8
food packaging, information on
   220
Freestyle Libre 291
fruit/veg common ground
   193–203

and anti-ageing antioxidants
195–6
best of 195
and fructose – in small
quantities 198–200
guidelines 202–3
and minimum daily portions
194
and polyphenol power 197–8
and skinny sirtuins 198
fruits, GL contained in 68
Fruitus Oat & Mixed Berry 257

G

G, K ad GKI, measuring 285–6,
296, 298
GABA 152
gamma-glutamyl transferase
(GGT) 16
Garry, Ann 77, 78, 79
Georgetown University Medical
Center 149
Gerber, Jeffry 37
glioblastomas, *see* neurogliomas/
glioblastomas
Global Energy Balance Network
(GEBN) 8
glucomannan fibre 224
glucose-dependent
insulinotrophic peptide
(GIP) 129
glucose with Freestyle Libre 291
glucose ketone 285–6
how to measure 286
glucose and ketone monitoring
in action 294–6
gluten 165, 167, 243
glycemic index (GI) (*see also*

high-fat, low-carb):
and food's quality 63
low, problems approach with
64–7
promoting foods with 61
and *quantity × quality* 64–5
and release of sugar 71
in tables 65, 66, 67
glycemic load (GL):
author champions 61
as better predictor 95
and blood-sugar level 71–3
and child's diets 114
and growth factors 107
and high diabetes 79–83
and low diabetes 75–6
low, improving heart health,
the evidence 97–100
and lowering blood pressure
101, 103
making sense? 83
and reducing blood pressure
and LDL 94, 98
and scientific studies 82
Slabber research 87
tips to lower 251
and Unwin 71–2
glycosylation 40, 95, 292–3, 299
goats 165–6
The Great Cholesterol Con
(Kendrick) 9
Great Ormond Street Hospital 56
Greeks 168

H

Hadza 164
haem iron 211
Harcombe, Zoe 5–6, 14, 21

Hardy, Karen 163
Harvard Medical School 82, 88,
    122, 174, 214
Harvard School of Public Health
    80, 82, 95, 106
  and cardiovascular risk
    declines 95
HbA1c 280, 292, 293
  and glucose levels 111
  as high measure of blood sugar
    75
  as key blood-sugar marker 19,
    20
  levels of predictor of 80
Health Professions Council of
    South Africa (HPCSA) 10–11
Hibbeln, Joseph 263
high-fat, low-carb (*see also*
    glycemic load):
  as answer 9
  and benefits of meal 44–5
  and blaming carbs 95–6
  delicious and varied 42
  and diets among patients with
    Parkinson's disease 57–8
  and Elliott 10
  and heart disease 35
  and heart disease and slow
    carbs 94–103
  and heart-disease strategy 40–1
  high-fat approach 44–5
  and high-fat diets 57
  and high-fat diets among
    patients with Parkinson's
    disease 57–8
  if flawed 6
  and insulin resistance 20, 39
  and issue of rebound weight
    gain 90–2

and less hunger 92–3
and losing weight 89
and low-carb approach 67–71
low carb with almost
    immediate remedy 114
and low carbs' meaning 22
and low GL in 219–24
and meal times 46
and metabolic advantage 91
and monitoring 47
more doctors join LC 61
nothing new in 43
and problems with latter 67–71
and quantity/quality
    combination 62
and reduced young death 35
and rising evidence 21
and severe epilepsy 24
for slow carb phase, *see* slow
    carb phase
three different energy sources,
    evidence for 45–6
UK recommendations of 15
and VLDL level 9
high-fat phase, for pescatarians,
    vegans and vegetarians
    266–7
high fat, phase of 217–33
  illustrated 218
  and importance of low GL in
    high-fat phase 219–20
  intake of 217–18
  sample menus 231–4
high-protein, high-fat veg 201–2
Holly, Jeff 213
Homo aquaticus 159–62
Homo sapiens 161, 163
Hong Kong 105
hooked on sugar 149–51

hormones, and different proteins 205

How to Lose Weight Well 177

how, why and when to switch 173–8

and dual-fuel timetable 176–7

and dynamics of fats, understanding 182

and working best 177–8

100% Health questionnaire 147, 194, 212

hunter-gatherer 131, 163

Hybrid Lattés 140, 141, 156, 175, 219, 227, 228, 232, 233, 297

hydroxybutyrate 184–5

hydroxycitric acid: the Thai secret 277–9

hyperinsulinemia 37

I

Ice Age 165

ideal glycosylated haemoglobin level 292–3

ideal protein needs 206–7

Imperial College London 30

inexorable rise of cancer 104–5 (*see also* cancer and high carbs)

Institute of Brain Chemistry and Human Nutrition 160

Institute for Optimum Nutrition 301

insulin:

balancing act 122–3

chromium reverses 280–1

plausibility of 35

raised 208

as true culprit 37–40

and worst memories 111

insulin-like growth factor (IGF-1) 31, 108, 124–5, 126, 215

insulin-resistant fat 20

intermittent fasting and exercise 137–45

and cardio and strength training 144

and fasting-mimicking diet 140–2

and intermittent fasting (IF) options 138–9

and interval training 143–4

need for 142–3

and words of caution 139–40

interval training 143–4

Ireland 111

Israel 161

Italy 99, 106–7, 108, 111

J

Jake 177

Japanese knotweed 32

Jenkins, David 61, 98, 209

Johns Hopkins University 29

Journal of Orthomolecular Medicine 88

Jubiz, William 273

K

Kalamian, Miriam 23–5

book by 25

Kalamian, Raffi 23–6

Kendrick, Malcolm 9, 36

Kenny, Paul 128, 130, 149, 150, 151

Keto for Cancer (Raffi) 25

ketone/glucose balance 284–99

ketone/glucose balance– *continued*
   in action 294–6
   G, K ad GKI 285–6
   and glucose and ketone
      monitoring in action 294–6
   and ideal glycosylated
      haemoglobin level 292–3
   ketosticks 288–9
   measuring 286, 289–90
   measuring ketones and glucose
      286
   and precise monitoring 296–9
ketone and glucose monitoring
   in action 294–6
ketone/ketogenic (*see also*
      ketone/glucose balance):
   advice on 46–7
   and counteract epilepsy 55–7
   babies run on 162
   diet right approach for all
      cancers? 32–3
   and diets, advice on 46–7
   diets, early days of 204
   difference between low GL and
      69–70
   glycosylated haemoglobin
      level, ideal 292–3
   and Harcombe 21
   inducing through starvation 18
   'keto flu' 46, 127
   Ketonix breath test 287–8
   from LG 174, 177
   and liver 287
   one of different energy sources
      45–6
   pioneers 17–19
   salts, in power form 189
   and side effects 56
   and slow carbs 151–2

start of diet of 132
and starvation response 18
starvation to initiate 21
synthetic, with MCT oil
   189–90
Ketonix 286–8, 295
Ketonix breath test 287–8
ketosticks 288–9
KEYA 290, 291
Keys, Ancel 4, 5, 34
King's College London 92–3
Korea 99
Kraft, Joseph 38
Krebs 279

L

L-dopa 57
lactic acid 121
lactose 63
Lancet 56
Lango, Valter 33
Larson, Joan Mathews 152
LCHF 10–11
LDL:
   and 'bad cholesterol' 9, 36, 185
   illustrated 182
Leader, Geoffrey 57–8
Leader, Lucida 57–8
Leicester, Roger 211
less hunger 92–3
Levine, John 157
LinkedIn 148
Longo, Valter 140–2, 144–5
low-carb, high-fat, *see* high-fat,
   low-carb
Ludwig Center 29
Ludwig, David 44–5, 122, 151, 174
lung cancer, one of top five 105

M

McDonald, Fiona 301
Maidenhead trial 77–9
  tables 77
maltose 63
Masai 164
Massachusetts Institute of
    Technology 124
Matthew's Friends Clinics 56
May, Theresa 291
'Mediterranean' diets 98
medium-chain triglyceride
    (MCT) 27, 51, 52, 53, 56, 182,
    189–90
  and high concentration of
    227

Menus: high-fat phase breakfasts:
  Chia or Walnut Coconut
      Yoghurt with Blueberries
      or Strawberries 308
  Hybrid Lattés 305–6
  Salmon with Asparagus
      Omelette 307
  Scrambled Egg with Smoked
      Salmon and Avocado
      306

Menus: high-fat phase main
    meals:
  Bangers and Cauliflower Mash
      314
  Cauliflower, Chickpea and Egg
      Curry 323–4
  Cauliflower Mash 324
  Cauliflower Rice 325
  Chicken Curry 320
  Chile con Carne 317–18

Creamy Salmon with Leeks
    322–3
Hummus Soufflé 313
Low Carb Kedgeree 311–13
Nick's Beefburgers 315–16
Pork Medallions with
    Watercress Salsa Verde
    321
Rib-eye Steak 316
Roasted Pepper Rolls with
    Goat's Cheese and Pine
    Nut Stuffing 319
Smoked Salmon with Crème
    Fraîche and Herb Sauce
    322
Spiced marinade 310–11
Spiced Turkey Burgers 314–15
Vegetarian Chilli 316–17

Menus: high-fat phase snacks:
  Goat's Cheese and Artichoke
      Pâté 308
  Gravadlax with Quail's Eggs
      310
  Guacamole 308
  Hummus and Egg Pâté 309

Menus: slow-carb breakfasts:
  Get Up & Go with CarboSlow®,
      Low Carb Milk and
      Berries 329
  Low GL Granola 331
  Oat and Chia Porridge 329
  Scrambled Eggs on Oatcakes
      or Pumpernickel 330
  Spiced Apples or Plums 330–1
  Yoghurt and Berries with
      Chopped Almonds 330

Menus: slow-carb main meals:
  Apple and Tuna Salad 334
  Beany Vegetable Soup 339
  Butternut Squash Salad 334–5
  Chestnut and Butter Bean
      Soup 340
  High Energy Lentil Soup 342–3
  Lentil and Lemon Soup 340–1
  Olive, Pine Nut and Feta Salad
      337–8
  Peruvian Quinoa Salad 336–7
  Quinoa Tabbouleh 338–9
  Salmon-Stuffed Avocado 336
  Spicy Pumpkin and Tofu Soup
      341–2
  Summer Pea and Mint Soup
      343–4
  Walnut and Three Bean Salad
      335–6

Menus: slow-carb other mains:
  Chickpea and Spinach Curry
      347–8
  Garlic Chilli Prawns with Pak
      Choi 348–9
  Kamut Spaghetti with
      Chestnut Mushrooms and
      Truffle Oil 345–6
  Thai Lamb Red Curry 346–7
  Trout with Puy Lentils and
      Roasted Tomatoes on the
      Vine 350–1
  Wholemeal Kamut Pasta with
      Borlotti Bolognese
      344–5

Menus: slow-carb snacks:
  Apple and Almond Cake
      333–4

  Low GL Carrot and Walnut
      Cake 331–3

Menus: what to drink:
  Alcohol 357–8
  Cold Drinks and Juices
      352–4
  Green and Black Tea 356
  Tea, Coffee and Chocolate
      354–6
Merck 37
Mesopotamia 165
metabolic syndrome 31, 55, 80,
      83, 111
metabolism, not calories 87–9
micronutrients, as efficient
      metabolism 271
micronutrients, as hybrid
      support 270–83
  amd carnitine 276–7
  and co-enzyme Q 274–6
  and elemental energy 279–80
  and energy nutrients 271–4
  and top mineral and tips
      282–3
milk, two proteins maintained
      by 213
Minnesota Coronary Experiment
      34–5
Minnesota University 153
mitochondria:
  and energy needed to function
      119
  extra source of fuel for 134
  and glucose 57
  and oxygen 29–30
  and vitamin B 48, 56
The Molecules of Emotion (Pert)
      149

monitoring diet (*see also* high-fat, low-carb), brain's need for 49–51
mood and memory from slow carbs 110–15
Mosley, Michael 140
mTOR 56, 113, 133, 134, 135, 174, 208, 215
  as body's fat controller 124–6, 142
  coffee suppresses 126
Mukherjee, Siddhartha 31–2

N

Nairn's oatcakes information 220–1
National Cancer Institute 214
National Institute for Health and Care Excellence (NICE) 17, 62
  and instruction to GPs 74
Nelofer, Syed 30
Netherlands 168
neurogliomas/glioblastomas 33, 104
neurotransmitters, and different proteins 205
new foods 166–7
Newport, Mary 49–51, 52–3
NHS:
  money saved on diabetes costs 15, 19
  and prediction by 2015 74
NICE, *see* National Institute for Health and Care Excellence
nicotinamide adenine dinucleotide (NAD) 48–9, 273–4

Nile Basin 165, 166
nitrosamines 211, 215
Noakes, Tim 10–11, 44
nomophobia 147
nutritional yoga 126–7

O

oatcakes 220–1
obese adolescents, at Harvard 82
oestrogens 106, 107
olive oil and oleic acid 184–5
omega-3:
  and DHA 159, 169
  enough for vegans 261–3
  how much needed? 263
  mainly in oily fish, nuts and seeds 14
  and poly-unsaturated 182–3
omega-6, and poly-unsaturated 182–3
oncologists' response 27–32
ORAC 195
Oregon Research Institute 150
overcoming resistance 20
Oxford University 194

P

paleo, vegan and ketogenic diets 168–71
Panasar, Arjun 19
pancreas cancer 29, 89
  one of top five 105
Panorama 155
Parkinson's disease 57–8, 134, 220
Parkinson's Disease (Leader, Leader) 58
Pawlak, Laura 89

Pereira, Maria 81, 91, 92
Pert, Candace 149
Peruvian Amazon 164
PET scans 23, 30
Pima Indians 167
polyphenol power 197–8
prescriptions 148
problem of dual fuel 127–8
prostate cancer:
   and dairy intake 214
   one of top five 105
protein, animal versus fish
    209–10
protein, not exceeding 204–16
   animal versus fish and
      vegetable protein 209–10
   the best of 210
   and dairy products and cancer
     213–14
   diabetes raised by 208
   enough from details – but not
     too much 215–16
   and exercise 214–15
   fat units 226–9
   fish 225–6
   ideal amounts 206
   and ideal protein needs 206–7
   and limiting carbs 229–30
   off meat 224–5
protein, problems with 263–4
proton pump inhibitors 273
Pureto Rican 111
pyruvate 29–30

Q

The Quest for Food (Crowe)
   165

R

Raffi's story on brain cancer
   23–6
randomised controlled trials
   (RCTs) 5
Reaven, Gerald 4
Rebel Kitchen 231
rebound weight gain, tackling
   90–2 (*see also* high-fat,
   low-carb)
red and processed meat and
   colorectal cancer 210–13
Ritalin 154
rogue gene mutations 23
Roman 168
ROS (reactive oxygen species) 31

S

Sabatini, David 124
St Joseph's Hospital 38
Samburu 164
sample menus 231–4, 257–9, 268–9
School of Medicine, Minnesota
   153
Sea of Galilee 165
serotonin 152
   and different proteins 205
Seven Weeks to Sobriety (Larson)
   152
Seyfried, Thomas 24, 278
Sherbrooke University 50
Silence of Peace (Levine) 157
skinny sirtuins 198
Slabber, Marthinete 87
slow carb phase 235–59, 264–6
   (*see also* high-fat, low-carb)
   baking 254–5

and beans and lentils 248–50
boiling 251, 253
cereal breakfasts 239–41
cooking methods 252–3
desserts 256–7
and eating for snacks 244–6
egg-and-toast breakfasts 242–3
fats and oils 252
and fishy breakfasts 244
fishy breakfasts 244
frying 255
and Get Up & Go breakfasts
    239
grilling 255
and lunch and dinner 246
microwaving 255
and more fish, less meat 246–7
and non-starchy vegetable
    250–1
plate illustrated 236, 238
poaching 254
sample menus 257–9
and snacks, what to eat for
    244–6
and starchy vegetable 247–8
steam frying 253–4
steaming 253
and tips to lower daily GL 251
and top tips for health cooking
    256
vegans in 264
vegetarian option 251–2
waterless cooking 254
and what to eat for breakfast
    236–8
when to eat 257
yoghurt breakfasts 241–2
snacks, what to eat for 244–6
Staples, Kate 144

starchy veg, avoiding 200–1
State University of Ceará 81
stomach cancer, one of top five
    105
sugar:
    and anger 113–14
    bitter truth about 62–4
    brain shrinkage by 113
    as cancer cause? 108–9
    common 63
    industry report 7
    'spoonful of . . .' 71–3
sugar, hooked on 149–51
suicide 146
supplements for energy 281–2
Sweden 106
Swiss Re 8
switching, why, when and how
    173–8
    and dual-fuel timetable 176–7
    and dynamics of fats,
        understanding 182
    and working best 177–8
synthetic ketones 189–90

T

tau 54
Teicholz, Nina 4–5, 11–12
Thai 167
Thailand 277–8
3–6–36 rule 79
thyroxine 154
Tofu Soup 266
top tips for healthy cooking 256
top vitamins and mineral tips
    282–3
Tripping over the Truth
    (Christofferson) 29

True Health Diagnostics 37
Trust Me, I'm a Doctor 140
tryptophan 152, 154
Tsimane 164
tyrosine 152, 154

U

UK studies 260
University of California 55, 108
University of Cape Town 44
University of East Anglia 262
University of Florida 151
University of Alabama Medical Center 272
University of Illinois 138
University of Southern California 33, 140
University of Sherbrook 162
University of Sydney 163
University of Texas 153
University of Toronto 61
Unwin, David 16–17, 22, 71, 76, 78–9, 83
  and different types of carbohydrate 17
  and low-carb 16
Unwin, Jen 79
Uruguay 161
US Government Anti-ageing Research Department 193
US studies 107, 111, 114, 260

V

Varady, Krista 138
Veech, Richard 50

vegans:
  enough omega-3 for 261–3
  and slow-carb phase 264–6
  UK number of 260
very low-density lipoproteins (VLDLs) 9 (*see also* LDL)
Virkkunen, Matti 114
vitamin B 48, 153, 169, 255, 261, 271–4, 280, 281
vitamin C 48, 88, 101, 153, 211, 239, 255, 271–4
vitamin D 12, 56, 169, 261
vitamins, and missing vitamins 169
vitamins and minerals, value of 55
Vogelstein, Bert 29
Volek, Geoff 4

W

Warburg, Otto 29
Watson, James 29
wheat, earliest 166
why, when and how to switch 173–8
  and dual-fuel timetable 176–7
  and dynamics of fats, understanding 182
  and working best 177–8
Willett, Walter 106
Williams, Matthew 27–8
Wise, Peter 31
Wiseman, Martin 211–12
Wokingham Medical Centre 76, 100
Wolever, Thomas 61
Wood, Susan 56

World Cancer Research Fund
    105, 106, 194, 211
World Health Organisation 194,
    212

Y

Yudkin, John 4

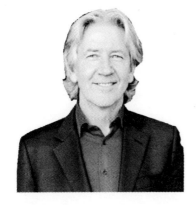

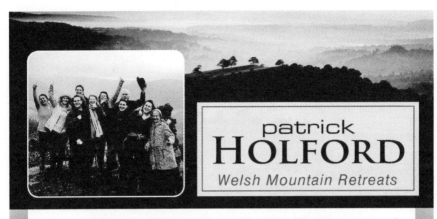